Peripheral Neuropathy

What It Is
and
What You Can Do to Feel Better

JANICE F. WIESMAN, MD

Johns Hopkins University Press

Baltimore

T0051427

Note to the reader: This book is not meant to substitute for medical care of people with neuropathy, and treatment should not be based solely on its contents. Instead, treatment must be developed in a dialogue between the individual and his or her physician. Our book has been written to help with that dialogue.

Drug dosage: The author and publisher have made reasonable efforts to determine that the selection of drugs discussed in this text conform to the practices of the general medical community. The medications described do not necessarily have specific approval by the U.S. Food and Drug Administration for use in the diseases for which they are recommended. In view of ongoing research, changes in governmental regulation, and the constant flow of information relating to drug therapy and drug reactions, the reader is urged to check the package insert of each drug for any change in indications and dosage and for warnings and precautions. This is particularly important when the recommended agent is a new and/or infrequently used drug.

© 2016 Johns Hopkins University Press
All rights reserved. Published 2016
Printed in the United States of America on acid-free paper
9 8 7 6 5 4 3 2

Johns Hopkins University Press
2715 North Charles Street
Baltimore, Maryland 21218
www.press.jhu.edu

Library of Congress Cataloging-in-Publication Data
Names: Wiesman, Janice F., 1958– author.
Title: Peripheral neuropathy : what it is and what you can do to feel better / Janice F. Wiesman, MD.
Description: Baltimore : Johns Hopkins University Press, [2016] | Series: A Johns Hopkins Press health book | Includes bibliographical references and index.
Identifiers: LCCN 2016002110| ISBN 9781421420844 (hardcover : alk. paper) | ISBN 1421420848 (hardcover : alk. paper) | ISBN 9781421420851 (paperback : alk. paper) | ISBN 1421420856 (paperback : alk. paper) | ISBN 9781421420868 (electronic) | ISBN 1421420864 (electronic)
Subjects: LCSH: Nerves, Peripheral. | Nerves, Peripheral—Diseases. | Health—Popular works.
Classification: LCC QP365.5 .W54 2016 | DDC 612.8/2—dc23 LC record available at http://lccn.loc.gov/2016002110

A catalog record for this book is available from the British Library.

Special discounts are available for bulk purchases of this book. For more information, please contact Special Sales at 410-516-6936 or specialsales@press.jhu.edu.

Contents

Preface   vii

1   What Is a Nerve?   1

2   What Is Neuropathy?   8

3   Symptoms of Neuropathy   15

4   Causes of Neuropathy   24

5   How Is Neuropathy Diagnosed?   38

6   Tests   46

7   Treatment of Neuropathy   64

8   Clinical Trials   86

9   Other Conditions That Feel Like Neuropathy   90

10   Living with Neuropathy   95

Acknowledgments   103
Glossary   105
References   109
Resources   111
Index   113

Preface

Approximately 20 million people in the United States have neuropathy. That is about 1 in every 15 persons. You may have neuropathy, and there is a good chance that you know other people who have neuropathy as well. This book is intended for you, and for them—and for your family members and professional caregivers. It explains nerves and neuropathy and describes what causes neuropathy as well as the symptoms. It walks the reader through the diagnosis and treatment of neuropathy and describes lifestyle changes that can help keep nerves healthy.

> I first heard the word "neuropathy" from my husband, who looked up my symptoms on the Internet. He said it meant nerve damage. He read to me all the symptoms and causes, and it seemed overwhelming. My primary doctor sent me to see a neurologist, who examined me, did some tests, and told me that I did have neuropathy. The tests showed that I also had early diabetes. The doctor said that high blood sugar, over a long time, can hurt the nerves, and that nerve injury causes the nerves to be activated when they shouldn't be. That is what was causing the tingling and pain. I was started on medicine and lost some weight, and my blood sugar went back to normal. After a few months, the tingling almost completely went away. I was on medicine to help with the pain, but I don't need that anymore.

This book is designed to take the reader through the same journey toward healing and symptom relief that my patients travel when I see them in the office. Over the past twenty years, I have gone through an abbreviated form of this book with patients individually and in small groups. When I speak at support group meetings for people who have neuropathy, inevitably someone approaches me and asks me to make my talk available. After pursuing this inefficient method of distribution for many years, I decided to listen to my patients and write this book. They have asked me for it.

This book is meant to be read in order from first chapter to last, and then to be used as a reference to look up specific topics. Basic definitions and concepts are discussed in the first few chapters; understanding these definitions and concepts is necessary for understanding the rest of the book. When appropriate, I refer the reader back to earlier chapters for a quick refresher and review. A glossary at the end of the book defines terms that may be unfamiliar to readers, and the resources section lists reliable websites and sources of additional information.

Peripheral Neuropathy

CHAPTER 1

What Is a Nerve?

What I want is muscles of iron and nerves of steel, inside
which dwells a mind of the same material as that of which the
thunderbolt is made.

Swami Vivekananda (1863–1902)

In popular use, the terms *nerve* or *nerves* refer to a person
feeling anxious or having a bold or unpleasant personality. People say, "I have a bad case of the nerves," or "He's so nervy," or "I
lost my nerve." That is not what this book is about. This book is
about harm to the anatomical structures called *nerves*. Nerves
are the electrical wiring of our bodies. Through nerves, our brain
receives information from the outside world. Nerves are also the
means by which our bodies act on the outside world.

Nerve cells, called *neurons*, are the cells in the body that make
up nerves. Each neuron has an armlike extension called an axon
that is surrounded by insulation called myelin (figure 1). A nerve
is a bundle of hundreds or thousands of axons that run in a connective tissue sheath (figure 2). Connective tissue is the material
that connects, binds, and supports the organs of the body.

The way neurons interact with each other is a true miracle of
nature. The neuron cell body is contacted by axons produced by
other neurons. Chemicals, called *neurotransmitters*, are released
from the end of the axon. The neurotransmitters cross a very
small space, called a *synapse*, to attach to specialized proteins,
called *receptors*, on the membrane that surrounds the neuron. A

neurotransmitter and receptor fit together like a key and lock. When the receptor is activated, an electrical impulse called an *action potential* travels down the axon membrane, like electricity down a wire, where it again causes the release of neurotransmitters. This continues along a chain of neurons that bring information from the outside world to the brain, and from the brain to the body. This sounds like a long, complicated sequence of events, but it all happens in a few thousandths of a second.

The nervous system is divided into the central nervous system and the peripheral nervous system. The central nervous system is made up of the brain and spinal cord. Nerve roots coming out of the spinal cord, nerves in the limbs and trunk, as well as the muscles make up the peripheral nervous system.

Neurons and their axons are divided into three functional categories: motor, sensory, and autonomic. Motor nerves run from the spinal cord outward to muscles and control voluntary movement. Sensory nerves bring sensations from skin, joints, and sense organs, like the eyes, ears, nose, and tongue, into the spinal cord and up to the brain. Autonomic nerves govern "automatic" functions like heart rate, body temperature, and movement of the gastrointestinal tract, among others.

There are two groups of motor neurons. One group is in the brain, and the other is in the spinal cord. Motor neurons in the brain are arranged anatomically in the cortex (outer surface) of the brain in the shape of a little person, called a *homunculus* (figure 3). The second group of motor neurons sits inside the spinal

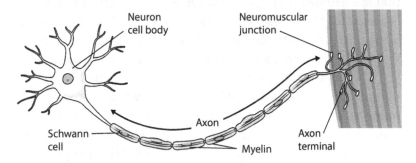

Figure 1 Nerve cell and neuromuscular junction

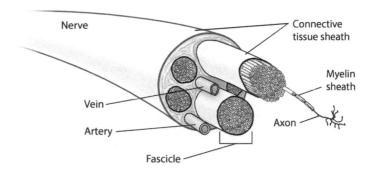

Labels on figure:
Nerve
Connective tissue sheath
Myelin sheath
Vein
Artery
Axon
Fascicle

Figure 2 Nerve

cord. Each motor neuron in the brain is "assigned" to control a certain muscle. A motor neuron in the brain sends an axon into the spinal cord, where it communicates with another motor neuron that is "assigned" to the same muscle. This second motor neuron sends an axon out of the spinal cord through its assigned nerve to its assigned muscle. Motor nerves bring information from the brain to the muscles to control voluntary movement. Neurotransmitters released by motor neurons at the synapse attach to receptors on muscle cells, which then make the muscle contract. We say that the nerve *innervates* the muscle.

There are also two groups of sensory neurons. Sensory neurons in the brain, like the motor neurons, are arranged like a homunculus (see figure 3). The second group is located not in the spinal cord, but in structures called *ganglia*, nerve tissue that forms a chain along both sides of the backbone (also called the *vertebral column*). Each sensory neuron in the ganglia sends out one axon that contacts sensory receptors in the skin and sense organs. Another, shorter extension (called a *dendrite*) is also sent out and enters the spinal cord. Sensory nerves bring information from specialized receptors in the skin, joints, and sense organs to the spinal cord. This information is then transmitted up the spinal cord to the brain.

Autonomic neurons sit both inside and outside the spinal cord, either close to the spinal cord or close to the organs they

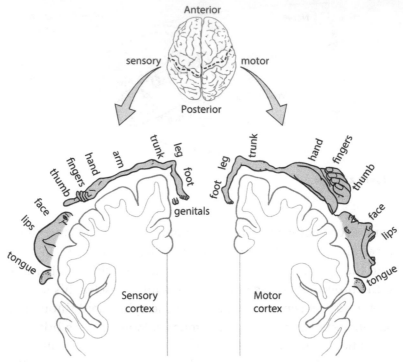

Figure 3 Motor and sensory homunculus

innervate. They monitor "automatic" functions, those we don't have to think about, like blood pressure and heart rate, and bring this information up to the brain. They also bring information from the brain out to the body to regulate automatic functions, including heart rate, blood pressure, body temperature, saliva and tear production, bowel movement, and sexual function.

Sensory nerves are organized like old-fashioned telephone lines. Each axon is "assigned" to a certain modality during fetal development. The assignment comes from the specialized sensory receptor in the skin that the nerve contacts. There are many different sensory receptors, and each has a name. For example, Pacinian corpuscles detect deep pressure and vibration, Meissner's corpuscles detect light touch, and free nerve endings detect pain and temperature. An axon that detects cold sensation on a certain small area of skin on the right big toe conducts its impulse to a certain small area of the spinal cord. The impulse then runs up the spinal cord in a specific area, ending in a specific part of the brain. Any impulse that comes from that specific axon and ends up in that specific part of the brain will be interpreted by the brain as "cold on the right big toe." So, in a sense, we do not "feel" with our skin or nerves; we feel with our brains. Likewise for the other senses: we see, hear, smell, and taste with our brains. The nerves from the eyes, ear, nose, and tongue are mere conduits for information from the outside world to the brain. The information is interpreted by the brain.

Sensory nerves emerge from the spinal cord as posterior (dorsal, or back) nerve roots. Motor nerves emerge from the spinal cord as anterior (ventral, or front) nerve roots (figures 4 and 5). Sensory and motor nerves merge with each other and with autonomic nerves to form the large named nerves that enter the arms, legs, and trunk. Most nerves contain axons from motor, sensory, and autonomic axons, but a few contain only one of the types. Different nerves go to different parts of the body in an orderly and consistent pattern. By knowing what part of the body is affected, your doctor will know which nerve or nerves are damaged.

In addition to being categorized by type, axons are also categorized by size. Autonomic axons are the thinnest, motor are the thickest, and sensory axons have a range of sizes from thin to thick. This is important for understanding the types of symptoms and the pattern of symptoms experienced by people with neuropathy.

Each axon is a thin and delicate structure, something that can be seen only under a microscope (figure 1). Axons are surrounded by a fatty coating, which is made by another type of cell called a Schwann cell. This fatty coating, called *myelin*, is much like the insulation of wires in a home in that it protects the nerve and insulates it from other axons. Myelin also makes the electrical impulse travel down the nerve faster. Very thin axons have an ultrathin myelin sheath and conduct their elec-

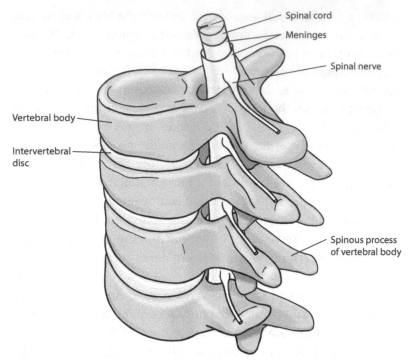

Figure 4 Spinal cord in the backbone

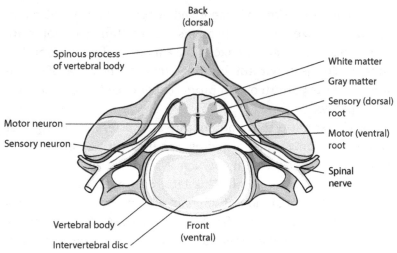

Figure 5 Spinal cord cross-section with motor and sensory roots

trical impulses slowly, at about 10 meters per second, or about 20 miles per hour. Axons with a much larger diameter and a thicker myelin coat conduct electricity at 60 meters per second, or about 130 miles per hour. In general, the autonomic axons are the thinnest, the motor axons are the thickest, and the sensory axons are in between.

Since the insulative coating on autonomic axons is thin, they are most susceptible to damage by toxins and mechanical forces, such as compression. Sensory axons are the next thickest group. The thinnest, most slowly conducting sensory axons bring information about pain and temperature from the skin to the spinal cord, where it is then transmitted up to the brain. Medium-sized sensory axons mediate touch. The thickest sensory axons, which conduct electricity most quickly, transmit information about deep pressure, vibration, and the position of joints. Motor axons are the thickest and conduct electricity the fastest.

The difference in conduction speed between the thinnest sensory axons and the thickest is noticeable in everyday life. A common experience is what you feel when you stub your toe. First you feel the stub, and then a split second later, you feel the pain. This is because the axons that transmit the pressure sensation of the "stub" conduct at 130 miles an hour, while the axons that transmit the pain conduct at only 20 miles an hour. The stub information gets to your brain faster than the pain information, so you feel the stub first and then the pain.

In later chapters, I describe how this anatomy explains the evolution of symptoms experienced by people with neuropathy. Some of the strange sensory symptoms of neuropathy can also be explained by the anatomy of nerves as described in this chapter.

CHAPTER 2

What Is Neuropathy?

On a good morning, I wake with most of my symptoms gone, except a persistent vibration in my feet and ankles that feels like numbness, even though I'm not numb. Neuropathy is tricky, because the symptoms don't make sense and often feel like something else. My symptoms are tied to the clock. The afternoon fatigue can be mind numbing. On most days, I experience a steady progression of vibration and electrical shocks extending up from my feet as well as a feeling like bugs are crawling on my skin. By afternoon, the neuropathic rheostat is turned up, and by dinner it is at full power, peaking when I try to sleep. My fingers and toes have a mind of their own, cramping and moving in directions I can't stop. In this condition, I sometimes find myself irritable, which is not a state I am used to. I work, I eat, I walk, I play with my grandchildren while in pain, and no one ever notices. My family, colleagues, and friends tell me I look well. Only my wife knows. It's a mystery to me, because I can be in a meeting where I feel like I will fall over, but I sip water, focus, and stay on point. Adrenaline and activity are friends. Finding balance is an ongoing challenge.

Neuropathy is a general term that refers to nerve damage. When one nerve is damaged, it is called *mononeuropathy*. Generalized damage to the nerves is called *polyneuropathy*, *peripheral neuropathy*, or simply *neuropathy*—the terms are interchangeable. Neuropathy itself is not usually a disease on its own but a symptom of an underlying illness. Sometimes that illness is obvious, other times not.

Types of Neuropathy

Most neuropathies, about 90 percent, involve damage to the axon itself. The surrounding fatty sheath, the myelin, is not affected. These are called *axonal neuropathies*. About 10 percent of the time, the damage is primarily to the myelin alone or in combination with damage to the axons. These are called *demyelinating neuropathies*. Some neuropathies are inherited and are not caused by an underlying illness. *Inherited neuropathies* can be the result of abnormalities of axons or myelin. Although this book focuses on axonal neuropathies, I would like to take a moment to discuss the other two types, as I refer to them in later parts of the book.

Demyelinating Neuropathy

As mentioned above, about 10 percent of neuropathies are caused primarily by damage to the myelin coating around the axon. Without this coating, the axon is vulnerable and can be damaged. These sorts of neuropathies typically arise from an attack on the myelin by the body's immune system. They are called *autoimmune neuropathies*. Autoimmune means that you make antibodies against what is actually a normal protein in your body.

Antibodies are large molecules made by white blood cells when those cells are exposed to a protein that is a threat to the body. In autoimmune disease, white blood cells make antibodies against proteins that are not actually threats. This can happen in two ways. The first is when white blood cells make an antibody specifically against a normal protein. The reasons this happens are not well understood. The second way is when an antibody is made against an infectious agent, like a virus or bacterium, which then cross-reacts with a similar-looking, normal protein in the body. This is called the *innocent bystander theory* of autoimmune disease. Most autoimmune neuropathies are demyelinating, primarily affecting the fatty coating around axons; rarely, they are axonal, primarily affecting the axons themselves.

A common form of the first mechanism is what can happen with bone marrow cancer. The bone marrow churns out too much of a certain antibody that attacks axons and myelin. The most common form of the second mechanism is called Guillain-Barré syndrome, also known as acute inflammatory demyelinating polyneuropathy. This typically happens after an infectious illness. There is controversy as to whether vaccinations or toxoid injections also cause this. Toxoids are chemically modified toxins that are made by bacteria. Toxoids are injected and used like a vaccine against the disease-causing toxin. Tetanus toxoid is a common example. Tetanus is a bacterium found in soil that produces a disease-causing toxin. If you get a deep cut or puncture wound that has dirt in it, your doctor may give you a tetanus toxoid injection to prevent the development of tetanus. Another form of the second mechanism is called chronic inflammatory demyelinating polyneuropathy. The cause is not as clear as it is for Guillain-Barré syndrome, but it causes damage in the same way. Guillain-Barré syndrome progresses over hours to a few weeks, and chronic inflammatory demyelinating polyneuropathy progresses over a few weeks to many months. In addition, other, very rare forms of demyelinating neuropathy are associated with specific antibodies. The diagnosis of such neuropathies involves blood tests for these antibodies.

Demyelinating neuropathy can also be caused by exposure to a toxin, such as that made by the diphtheria bacterium or the toxin found in buckthorn berries. Medications can cause this neuropathy as well, including chloroquine, tacrolimus, perhexiline, procainamide, and zimelidine.

The steps to diagnosis are the same as those for axonal neuropathy, which I discuss later in the book. Diagnosis is important because treatment can shorten the course of demyelinating neuropathy and prevent long-term disability. These treatments include medicines that suppress the immune system, such as steroids; intravenous immunoglobulin; and drugs that are also used in the treatment of cancer. A procedure called *plasma exchange* is sometimes used. In this procedure, small amounts of blood are removed, and the red blood cells are separated from the plasma. The red cells are then returned to the body, while the plasma, which contains the antibodies, is discarded. Plasma exchange can be thought of as a blood-cleaning procedure. The discarded plasma is replaced with the protein albumin, which comes from donated blood.

Inherited Neuropathy

Inherited neuropathies are all caused by genetic mutations that are passed down in families. Our genes are passed down in chromosomes. We have twenty-three pairs of chromosomes: one pair of sex chromosomes, and twenty-two pairs called *autosomal* chromosomes. Genetic mutations can affect genes on the sex chromosomes or on the autosomal chromosomes.

There are many different types of inherited neuropathy, each the result of a different genetic mutation. It is important to distinguish between genetic mutations that directly cause nerves or their myelin to develop abnormally and mutations that cause a disease that then leads to neuropathy. In this section, I discuss the former: inherited disorders of axons and myelin.

In some inherited disorders, a family history is obvious; in others, it is not. The most common type of inherited neuropathy is the result of abnormal production of myelin. Symptoms often start in childhood, when the child has difficulty walking and running. Inherited neuropathies are typically not painful, but they do cause weakness. If neuropathy starts at a young age, with a family history of such problems, genetic testing may be useful (this is discussed in chapter 6).

The most common directly inherited neuropathy is Charcot-Marie-Tooth disease type 1 (also called hereditary sensory-motor neuropathy type 1). It is named after the three physicians who first described it more than one hundred years ago. This neuropathy is inherited in an autosomal dominant fashion, meaning that only one copy of the mutated gene is needed to cause disease. For each gene, you have two copies, one from your mother and one from your father. Typically, with an autosomal dominant neuropathy, one parent has also had symptoms. Each child of that parent has a 50 percent chance of getting the mutated gene and hence the neuropathy. When neuropathy is inherited in this way, the family history is often obvious. In Charcot-Marie-Tooth disease type 1, the mutation is in the PMP22 gene, which governs the manufacture of a certain protein in myelin. The mutation causes production of myelin that is thinner than it should be, with an abnormal chemical composition. The myelin works, but not as well as normal myelin. Other autosomal dominant gene mutations lead to the production of abnormal myelin, but they are less common.

Other inherited neuropathies have an autosomal recessive pattern of inheritance, meaning that you need to inherit two copies of the mutated gene for the disease to occur. A person with only one copy of the mutated gene will not have the disease. When both parents have one copy of the mutated gene, each child has a 25 percent chance of receiving both mutated genes. Some neuropathies have an X-linked pattern of inheritance, meaning the mutation is on the X chromosome. These neuropathies affect only males, who have one X and one Y chromosome. Females have two X chromosomes, so if one X has the mutation, they still have the normal gene on the other X chromosome. In these forms of inheritance, a family history may not be obvious.

Axonal Neuropathy

This book focuses on axonal neuropathies. Axonal neuropathies have the same pattern of symptoms and examination findings regardless of the cause. They are called *axonal, length-dependent, dying-back neuropathies*. This phrase gives a lot of information about what is going on. Axonal means that the axon itself is affected, rather than the fatty insulation. Length dependent means that the longest nerves are affected first. Dying back (an unfortunate phrase) means that the nerves degenerate from the ends up. What explains this pattern?

The pattern is easy to understand when you think about where the axons come from. As described in chapter 1, axons are armlike projections of the neuron. The cell body of the neuron makes structural proteins and energy-containing molecules that are transported from the cell body to the end of the axon. The cell body also contains tiny organs that absorb waste products made by the axon. Blood brings energy-containing molecules from food to the cells, and when these molecules are used, waste products are formed, which can be toxic to the cell. The axon transports the waste products back to the cell body, which neutralizes them. Throughout the neuron's lifetime, the cell body must make new parts for the axon and clear the waste products of metabolism. A neuron is about 50 microns (millionths of a meter) wide, and it has to support the metabolism of an arm that could be 3 feet long. That is like a person who is 6 feet tall having an arm that is 20 miles long! The neurons that make the nerves do not regenerate; you do not make new ones. The neurons you are born with are expected to do their job for 120 years. With all this responsibility, it is easy to see how just a little bit of damage to a neuron would make it unable to properly support its axon. Because important proteins made in the neuron cell body have to travel all the way down to the end of the axon, the end is the most vulnerable portion. It is the first to degenerate when the neuron is sick.

In neuropathy, nerves degenerate from the end back up toward the spinal cord. I am often asked if nerves can grow back. Nerve regeneration is iffy. Under the best conditions, they grow at a rate of about one millimeter a day. This translates into one inch per month and one foot per year. As we get older and develop different illnesses, however, regrowth is less successful. No medications can help nerves regrow. The goals of treating axonal neuropathies are to address the underlying cause, if possible; treat the symptoms; and improve function. We then try not to cause further harm while waiting to see if the nerves regenerate.

In axonal neuropathy, another common pattern is that the thinnest axons tend to be affected first, with the thickest affected later on. There are many reasons for this pattern, known and unknown. What it means is that often people with neuropathy first notice autonomic dysfunction (such as lightheadedness due to low blood pressure, dry mouth, and erectile dysfunction), pain, and loss of the ability to feel temperature. Later, they notice loss of joint position sense as well as muscle weakness.

Most axonal neuropathies start insidiously, with barely noticeable symptoms, and progress over many months to years to the point where a person with these symptoms will seek medical attention. Infrequently, axonal neuropathies that are caused by malnutrition, medication, or rare immunological problems can progress quickly.

Some causes of axonal neuropathy do not obey the "length-dependent" rule, including neuropathy caused by some anticancer medications, vitamin B12 deficiency, or overuse of vitamin B6. Common and uncommon causes of neuropathy are discussed in chapter 4.

CHAPTER 3

Symptoms of Neuropathy

I first knew something was wrong when I retired and had time to play three or four rounds of golf weekly. I noticed a decline in my golf game and developed a lot of fatigue in my legs while walking the course and climbing stairs to the pro shop. From fatigue in my legs, I moved on to muscle cramping and twitching of my calf muscles, then numbness and tingling of my fingers. Over the next year, I gradually began losing strength in my arms and legs on both sides, and I started feeling a burning, electrical shock–type pain in my hands, along with a sensation of coldness. My fingers would feel stiff and weak, which made it hard for me to button or zip my clothes or to hold a glass. To accept my limitations, I now focus on the things I can do and not what I can't do. I stay as active as possible. I walk the treadmill at the gym, work in my garden, and just keep moving!

Sensory Symptoms

Sensory symptoms are often among the first and most bothersome symptoms of neuropathy. Doctors categorize symptoms as *positive*, meaning noticeable sensations, and *negative*, meaning lack of sensation. Positive sensations include pain and tingling; numbness is a negative symptom.

When doctors think about sensory symptoms, they divide them into symptoms mediated by small axons and those mediated by large axons. Small-axon symptoms include tingling, burning, shooting or electrical pain, itching, buzzing, a feeling as though ants are crawling on the skin, and an increased sensitivity of the skin. Normal stimulation of the skin, such as a light touch of clothing or bedsheets on the legs, can feel uncomfortable or painful. Large axon symptoms include numbness, stiffness, squeezing, and feeling off balance.

The feeling of poor coordination, or being off balance, comes from loss of sensation in the joints of the feet and ankles. Normally, this information is brought up to the brain, and we register the sensation without thinking about it. When this information is lost, the brain does not know where the toes and feet are in space, which makes you feel off balance. Then, to maintain your balance, you have to look to see where you are.

The length-dependent nature of neuropathy explains the physical pattern of symptoms. Pain, tingling, and electrical sensations start in the soles of the feet and in the toes, which are at the end of the longest nerves, slowly moving up to the ankle and leg. When symptoms reach the knee, the hands will then become involved because the nerves to the hands are the same length as those to the knees. In some types of neuropathy, particularly those caused by medication, taste is less intense or different. Taste buds are simply specialized nerve endings, and if they are damaged by medication, they usually regenerate within a few weeks after the drug is stopped.

People with neuropathy wonder how their feet can feel numb and painful at the same time. The answer lies in the different functions of the various sensory nerve types. When the small axons are damaged, they tend to fire off impulses randomly; because of the connections between the nerve, spinal cord, and brain, these firings are interpreted by the brain as pain and tingling. When the large axons are damaged, they do not provide the brain with information, and this loss is interpreted by the brain as numbness.

Motor Symptoms

Neuropathy can cause muscle weakness. This is different from the general weakness that people feel when they are tired.

Neuropathy causes a specific weakness of some muscles and not others. The nerves that run from the spinal cord to the muscles are called *motor nerves*. They are thicker in diameter than sensory nerves and are covered with a thicker coat of myelin. These two characteristics make motor nerves less susceptible to damage. Motor symptoms typically appear later than sensory symptoms. In addition, the weak muscles may also become smaller, what doctors call *atrophy*.

Each motor axon branches to innervate dozens to thousands of muscle cells. Weakness occurs because some axons have degenerated and some are not functioning properly. Too few working axons are left to stimulate enough cells in each muscle to make the muscle contract with full power. Atrophy occurs because the muscle depends on nerve stimulation to stay healthy. Nerve endings typically release growth factors in addition to releasing neurotransmitters. With neuropathy, there are fewer nerve endings to do this, and the muscle becomes smaller.

Early symptoms include tripping over one's toes and trouble standing on heels and toes. As neuropathy progresses, weakness can include difficulty walking up stairs and getting out of a chair. Because neuropathy is length dependent, by the time weakness affects the muscles of the thigh, it has started in the hands. Early symptoms in the hands include trouble picking up small objects (like coins) and difficulty holding onto objects like utensils or a coffee cup.

Damage to motor nerves can also cause muscle cramps, *fasciculations* (muscle twitching), swelling in the legs, and foot deformity. Muscle cramps can affect small or large muscles and can be quite painful. They are more common at night. Even though cramps are a frequent symptom of neuropathy, the cause is not completely understood. Fasciculations feel like tiny jumping or twitching muscles under the skin. They are caused by sick motor neurons that fire impulses at random.

When muscles in the legs are weak, they don't act as they should to pump blood up from the legs to the body, so swelling, or *edema*, can develop. In long-standing neuropathy, deformities of the foot can occur. Weakness of the small muscles of the foot prevent them from holding the bones of the foot in proper alignment.

Distinguishing between weakness and loss of sensation is important. With loss of sensation, it is difficult to know how firmly the hand is gripping an object, and it can seem like weakness when an object falls from a numb hand. Another important distinction is between neuropathy affecting the hands in general and carpal tunnel syndrome, where one specific nerve is compressed in the wrist, leading to weakness of a certain group of muscles in the hand. See chapter 9 for more details about carpal tunnel syndrome.

Autonomic Symptoms

The autonomic part of the nervous system refers to the functions of the body that are not under voluntary control. This less-known but significant part of the nervous system controls vital functions of the body:

- Blood pressure and heart rate (how fast the heart beats)
- Regulation of blood flow to the hands and feet
- Saliva manufacture by the salivary glands in the mouth
- Tear manufacture by the lacrimal glands in the eyes
- Sweat production by sweat glands in the skin
- Skin and nail lubrication
- Vision function, including adjustment of the pupil to allow more or less light to enter the eye and adjustment of the lens of the eye to allow focus on far or near objects
- Emptying of the bladder
- Movement of the bowel
- Sexual function

Autonomic symptoms of neuropathy include lightheadedness, cold feet and hands, dry mouth and eyes, sweating changes, dry skin, hair loss on the arms and legs, brittle nails, vision changes, bladder dysfunction, various digestive tract problems, sexual dysfunction, and loss of the body's ability to detect low blood sugar and even heart attack.

Lightheadedness

Normally, when you stand up from lying flat or sitting, your blood pressure falls for a short time and then increases to just above normal. Autonomic nerves supply both the heart and the muscles in the walls of arteries. Arteries are the blood vessels that bring blood from the heart to the organs of the body, including the brain. When the autonomic nervous system detects a drop in blood pressure, it compensates in two ways. The first is constriction of arteries, making them narrower and increasing the pressure of the blood inside them. The second is stimulation of the heart to increase the heart rate, which will also increase blood pressure. If these mechanisms are insufficient to raise blood pressure enough to pump blood to the brain, gravity takes over and pulls the blood down into the legs. This leads to a feeling of lightheadedness. Symptoms of lightheadedness with prolonged standing, walking, or exercise can be due to loss of these compensatory mechanisms. This is a particularly dangerous problem in that it can lead to fainting and falls, which cause injury. Straining while having a bowel movement or urinating can also lower blood pressure and cause lightheadedness. Feeling lightheaded can also be the result of dehydration or an abnormal heart rate or rhythm. Your doctor can test for these causes.

Cold Feet and Hands

Autonomic nerves innervate the small muscles in the walls of arteries. These nerves can make the arteries dilate (widen), increasing blood flow, or constrict (narrow), decreasing blood flow. Blood flow to the hands and feet make them feel warm. With autonomic neuropathy, sometimes blood flow is restricted, causing hands and feet to feel cold.

Dry Mouth

Saliva is made in the salivary glands in the mouth. It wets the mouth and contains enzymes that start the digestion of food. The thought, sight, and smell of food makes the glands active in anticipation of eating. Autonomic nerves stimulate the salivary glands, causing them to produce saliva. If the nerves are few in number or are not working well, saliva production will decrease, resulting in a dry mouth. In addition to feeling uncomfortable, dry mouth can lead to problems with swallowing as well as cavities and growth of bacteria in the mouth.

Dry Eyes

As with saliva production, the autonomic nerves supply the lacrimal glands in the eyes to stimulate tear production. Dry eyes are uncomfortable and increase the risk of infection and scratches of the cornea.

Changes in Sweating

Sweat production is regulated by autonomic nerves that innervate sweat glands in the skin. Sweating is important in regulating body temperature. With neuropathy, decreased sweating is noted in the legs, and sometimes increased compensatory sweating is felt in other areas of the body. This can lead to feelings of heat intolerance and increased sweating in the face, back, and underarms.

Changes in Skin and Nails

Autonomic nerves supply sebaceous glands, which sit inside hair follicles in the skin. These glands produce oil (sebum) that lubricates the skin and hair. Loss of these nerves leads to dry, thin skin and hair loss. Nails are a type of specialized skin, and with neuropathy, nails can become ridged and brittle.

Vision Symptoms

The pupil of the eye is much like the aperture of a camera. It is made of a sphincter muscle called the iris (the colored part of the eye). A *sphincter* is a cylindrical muscle. When a sphincter muscle contracts, the opening in the middle of the cylinder gets smaller, and when it relaxes, the opening gets bigger. There are many sphincter muscles throughout the body, and most regulate the movement of substances from one part of the body to another. The iris opens and closes to regulate the amount of light entering the eye. This muscle contraction is governed by autonomic nerves. In neuropathy, it may be difficult for the eyes to adjust to changes in ambient light.

The lens is a soft sphere that sits inside the eye and focuses images projected onto the back of the eye. Tiny muscles contract to pull the lens thinner so that close-up images are in focus. When they relax to let the lens ball up, distant images are in focus. Autonomic nerves innervate these small muscles. When they are not working well, the lens cannot change shape as it should, and images, particularly close ones, will be out of focus.

Bladder Dysfunction

The bladder is essentially a bag lined with muscle, with a sphincter muscle at the bottom to regulate the outflow of urine. Sensory nerve endings are present in the wall of the bladder. Stretching of these nerve endings signals bladder fullness. Motor nerves cause contraction of the bladder. Neuropathy can lead to loss of bladder fullness sensations, difficulty contracting the bladder, and incoordination of sphincter relaxation and bladder wall contraction to allow the passage of urine from the bladder. Straining to urinate, difficulty in starting the stream of urine, and weakness of the stream are common symptoms. When the bladder is not completely emptied, urine is stored there, with stretching of the bladder wall. This can, in turn, cause overflow leakage of urine and increased risk of infection of the urine that is held in the bladder. This happens slowly, over time. People are often not aware of bladder dysfunction until they have a urinary tract infection.

Movement of the Digestive Tract

The esophagus, stomach, and small and large intestines contain in their walls approximately 100 million nerve cells under the control of the autonomic nervous system. If that system is not working correctly, the esophagus will not propel food from the throat into the stomach, giving a feeling of something being caught in the throat. The stomach will not empty as it should, so food will remain in the stomach for too long, causing a feeling of fullness, nausea, or abdominal pain after eating even a small meal. Autonomic dysfunction can cause the bowel to be overactive or underactive, resulting in diarrhea or constipation. Some people may alternate between the two. Long-standing diarrhea can lead to malnutrition. Autonomic nerves also supply the anal sphincter muscle at the end of the large intestine. Weakness of this muscle can lead to incontinence of stool.

Sexual Dysfunction

Sexual dysfunction is a common problem early on with autonomic neuropathy. Autonomic nerves stimulate the blood vessels in the penis and in the clitoris to dilate and fill with blood, leading to erection of the penis and engorgement of the clitoris. Autonomic nerves also stimulate glands in the vagina to produce lubricating fluid. Autonomic neuropathy can cause erectile dysfunction in men and decreased vaginal lubrication in women. It can interfere with the ability to achieve orgasm in both sexes.

Detection of Low Blood Sugar

The autonomic nervous system detects low blood sugar, signaling the condition by producing symptoms such as sweating, shakiness, nausea, headache, fast heart rate, and a feeling of anxiety. In diabetes, the use of medication to lower blood sugar along with decreased food intake can lead to low blood sugar levels, called *hypoglycemia*. In those with autonomic dysfunction, the normal alert system does not work, and low blood sugar can go undetected.

Silent Heart Attack

Autonomic nerves signal pain during a heart attack. Coronary blood vessels supply the heart itself with blood. In a heart attack, a blocked coronary artery deprives part of the heart of blood, causing pain. With autonomic dysfunction, this pain may not be felt, and a heart attack not detected.

CHAPTER 4

Causes of Neuropathy

For most diagnoses all that is needed is an ounce of knowledge, an ounce of intelligence, and a pound of thoroughness.

Arabic proverb

This chapter explores the many causes of neuropathy. Nerve damage can be due to disease, medications, toxins, alcohol use, and vitamin deficiencies or overuse. People who already have some neuropathy will be more severely affected when faced with a second cause of neuropathy than someone who has never had it before. Rarely, neuropathy is an illness unto itself and is inherited.

Neuropathy Associated with Illness

Neuropathy is a symptom of many illnesses. Some are inherited, and others occur out of the blue. In the United States, the most common cause is diabetes mellitus, but neuropathy can occur even with *prediabetes*, also called *glucose intolerance*. There are hundreds of causes of neuropathy. Table 4.1 lists some of the more well-documented causes. This table includes axonal, demyelinating, and inherited neuropathies.

How the nerves are damaged varies in different diseases, but common mechanisms include:

- Toxic effect on the nerve cell body, the axon, or the myelin coating, as can be seen with some anticancer drugs and antibiotics

- Interference with the transport of substances from the cell body to the end of the axon, as can be caused by some anticancer medications
- Physical compression of axons, for example, by deposits of insoluble proteins in the sheath of connective tissue that surrounds nerves, as is seen in amyloidosis
- Inflammation of the blood vessels that supply the nerves, leading to small "strokes" of the nerves, as can be seen in rheumatologic diseases such as rheumatoid arthritis and systemic lupus erythematosus

A Word about Diabetes Mellitus

Until recently, leprosy was the most common cause of neuropathy in the world. It has recently been surpassed as the number one cause by diabetes, which leads to neuropathy in many people. There are two types of diabetes, type 1 and type 2. Type 1, which is far less common, is also called juvenile diabetes, because it comes on in childhood. It is probably caused by an autoimmune attack on the cells in the pancreas, called islet cells, that produce insulin in response to the glucose (sugar) level in the blood. Type 2 is by far the more common type, and it is increasing throughout the world. Both types of diabetes can cause neuropathy.

At some point in the course of their illness, 50 percent of people with diabetes will develop neuropathy. The longer a person is diabetic, the more likely he is to have neuropathy. At the time of diagnosis, 20 percent of people will already have neuropathy. This tells us that nerve damage starts before the diagnosis is made and before people have symptoms that bring them to the doctor. Sometimes, neuropathy is the first symptom of diabetes. In recent years, the concept of *prediabetes* has been recognized. In prediabetes, blood glucose is not high enough to establish a diagnosis of diabetes mellitus, but it is higher than normal. A normal fasting glucose level is less than 100 mg/dl (milligrams per deciliter), while a fasting level of greater than

Table 4.1 Causes of Neuropathy

Metabolic illness that is not inherited
    Diabetes mellitus
    Malnutrition
    Vitamin B1, B6, B12, or E deficiency or toxicity
    Celiac disease
    Connective tissue diseases
        Systemic lupus erythematosus
        Rheumatoid arthritis
        Mixed connective tissue disease
        Sjögren's syndrome
    Kidney disease (uremic neuropathy)
    Hypothyroidism
    Primary amyloidosis
Metabolic illness that is inherited
    Porphyria
    Pompe disease
    Fabry disease
    Familial amyloidosis
    Friedreich's ataxia
    Adrenomyeloneuropathy
Infectious illness
    Human immunodeficiency virus
    Hepatitis C
    Diphtheria
    Leprosy
Postinfectious/autoimmune disorders
    Guillain-Barré syndrome
    Chronic inflammatory demyelinating polyneuropathy
    Acute axonal neuropathy
Medication side effect
Toxins
Treatment in the Intensive Care Unit
Cancer
    Primary amyloidosis
    Paraneoplastic neuropathy
    Radiation treatment
Damage to the blood supply
Inherited neuropathies
    Hereditary motor and sensory neuropathy (many types)
    Hereditary neuropathy with liability to pressure palsies

126 mg/dl is diagnostic of diabetes. People with fasting glucose levels between 100 and 125 fall into the category of prediabetes. Another common test to look at glucose in the blood is called *hemoglobin A1c*. Hemoglobin is the iron-containing protein in red blood cells that carries oxygen. The results of the hemoglobin A1c test reflect the percentage of hemoglobin that has glucose attached to it. A normal level is less than 5.7 percent. In diabetes, it is greater than 6.5 percent. Between 5.7 and 6.4 percent lies prediabetes.

There are many theories about how diabetes causes neuropathy. Multiple effects of elevated blood glucose, as found in diabetes, are likely causes of nerve damage. One effect is on blood vessels. Diabetes damages the blood vessels that bring oxygen and nutrients to neurons and to the cells that make myelin. Extra glucose in cells will attach to proteins and change their function. A byproduct of sugar metabolism called *sorbitol* may also damage nerves in two ways: (1) by inhibiting the formation of energy-containing molecules that cells need to function, and (2) by increasing the amount of a destructive form of oxygen called a *free radical*, which damages membranes like the one that envelops neuron cell bodies and their axons. People with diabetes often have elevated levels of triglycerides, a type of fat, in the blood. High levels of triglycerides are also associated with the development of neuropathy. Finally, people with diabetes who smoke are at increased risk of developing neuropathy.

Rarely, some people with very high blood sugars experience the sudden onset of painful sensory neuropathy after treatment is started and blood sugar is lowered. This condition is called *treatment-related neuropathy*. Typically a transient problem, treatment-related neuropathy resolves when good blood sugar control is maintained. The cause is not known. Both pain and autonomic dysfunction can occur without weakness.

Malnutrition

Neuropathy can be caused by nutritional deficiencies. Illnesses that interfere with absorption of food from the stomach and intestine, prolonged periods of being unable to eat or being fed intravenously, and weight-loss surgery (bariatric surgery) are the most common causes of this sort of neuropathy.

Vitamin and Mineral Deficiency and Toxicity

Vitamins are coenzymes, organic molecules that work with enzymes in the body to speed up chemical reactions involved in just about every aspect of metabolism. Enzymes are proteins that accelerate chemical reactions in the body. Some vitamins cannot be made by the human body and must be eaten in the diet. Deficiency of vitamins B1, B6, B12, and E can cause damage to nerves.

Deficiency of vitamin B12 (also called cyanocobalamin) is the most common vitamin deficiency to cause neuropathy. Symptoms include pain that starts in the hands and feet at about the same time, breaking the rule about starting first in the feet. This vitamin is necessary for myelin formation. Without it, myelin production decreases, which leads to less protection for axons and a greater risk of damage. Vitamin B12 is found in meat and eggs. Those on a strict vegetarian or vegan diet may require B12 supplementation. To be absorbed, vitamin B12 requires stomach acid as well as help from another protein called *intrinsic factor*. This protein is made by cells in a particular part of the stomach, cells that can be damaged by ulcers or inflammation of the stomach. *Pernicious anemia* is a disorder in which intrinsic factor is not available, because of damage to the cells that make it or the presence of antibodies against the factor itself. Pernicious anemia has many causes. As people get older, they make less acid in the stomach, which interferes with B12 absorption. An increasingly common cause of vitamin B12 deficiency is weight-loss surgery that includes removing the part of the stomach that produces intrinsic factor.

Vitamin B1 (thiamine) deficiency can cause a painful neuropathy as part of a condition called *beriberi*, from the Sinhalese word for weakness. Thiamine is found in brown rice, grains, and meat. B1 deficiency from poor diet is common with heavy alcohol use.

Vitamin B6 (pyridoxine) deficiency can cause a painful neuropathy that starts in the hands and feet at the same time, again breaking our usual rule. This vitamin is found in many foods, including fish, poultry, seeds, nuts, and fortified grains and cereals. Two medications—hydralazine, for high blood pressure, and isoniazid, for tuberculosis—cause increased excretion of vitamin B6, which can lead to neuropathy through B6 deficiency. Too much vitamin B6, however, can also lead to neuropathy. At a dose greater than 100 mg (milligrams) a day, B6 can damage sensory neurons, causing them to have trouble maintaining their long axons. This leads to a painful sensory neuropathy.

Vitamin E (tocopherol) deficiency causes neuropathy characterized by incoordination, trouble with balance, and weakness. Vitamin E is found in nuts, seeds, and vegetable oils.

Very rarely, decreased copper levels can cause neuropathy. This is sometimes the result of a high intake of zinc, sometimes in the form of zinc-containing denture adhesive, which causes decreased copper absorption in the intestine.

Celiac Disease

People with celiac disease (gluten-sensitive enteropathy), defined by the presence of antibodies to a wheat protein called *gliadin*, may develop an axonal neuropathy. The exact mechanism that causes nerve damage is not known but may be related to inflammation caused by antibodies to gliadin.

Connective Tissue Diseases

Connective tissue diseases are diseases of collagen and elastin, proteins that bind together the structures of the body. Connective tissue sits under the skin and makes up tendons, ligaments, and the sheaths that surround nerves, among other structures. A few connective tissue diseases are associated with neuropathy, including systemic lupus erythematosus, rheumatoid arthritis, mixed connective tissue disease, and Sjögren's syndrome. Sjögren's syndrome, an autoimmune disorder, leads to destruction of sensory neurons in the dorsal root ganglia (the groups of sensory neurons that sit inside the dorsal root as it emerges from the spinal cord) and typically causes a painful neuropathy. The cause of neuropathy in these disorders is not completely understood but may be related to damage of small blood vessels.

Neuropathy While in an Intensive Care Unit

Patients in an Intensive Care Unit (ICU) are quite ill and require intensive treatment. Their illnesses and their treatments can both cause neuropathy. Multiple organ failure leaves the body unable to get rid of normally produced toxins, an accumulation that can cause neuropathy. Patients in the ICU often cannot eat on their own and must be fed intravenously. This method of feeding cannot replace all the nutrients in food and, if prolonged, can lead, paradoxically, to neuropathy due to malnutrition. Some of the medications used in the ICU can also cause neuropathy.

Kidney Disease

Chronic kidney disease (also called *renal insufficiency*) can, over the long term, result in neuropathy, even in people who do not require dialysis. The kidneys filter waste products from the blood, and the buildup of these waste products can cause what's called *uremic neuropathy*. Even those with kidney failure who are on dialysis can develop neuropathy because dialysis is imperfect and does not remove waste products with the same efficiency as a kidney.

Hypothyroidism

Hypothyroidism is characterized by a low thyroid hormone level, which can, over time, lead to neuropathy. This is rare given the severe degree of thyroid dysfunction required to cause nerve damage.

A Word about Amyloidosis

Amyloidosis is an under-recognized cause of neuropathy. It is rare, and many physicians have never seen it. The word *amyloidosis* refers to deposits of an insoluble protein in many organs of the body, including in the nerves. (Insoluble means it is difficult if not impossible to dissolve in liquid.) The protein may be an inherited abnormal version of a protein made in the liver called *transthyretin*, a protein made by cancer cells in the bone marrow, or other proteins related to chronic illness. The first symptoms are autonomic dysfunction and pain. Neuropathic symptoms often start months to years before a diagnosis is made. (I discuss steps to diagnosis in chapter 5.) If you have symptoms of neuropathy and a cause is not found, consider amyloidosis.

Inherited Metabolic Illness

A wide variety of inherited metabolic illnesses can have neuropathy as a symptom, often a minor symptom. These disorders are rare and include porphyria, Pompe disease, Fabry disease, familial amyloidosis, Friedreich's ataxia, and adreno-myeloneuropathy.

Infectious and Postinfectious Causes of Neuropathy

Infection can cause neuropathy, either directly, by means of a toxin made by the infectant, or indirectly, by the body's response to an infectious agent. Postinfectious neuropathies are caused when the immune system makes antibodies to an infectious agent that then cross-react with normal proteins on the axon membrane or on the myelin.

Infections that can cause neuropathy include hepatitis C, human immunodeficiency virus (HIV), and leprosy, caused by the bacterium *Mycobacterium leprae*. Until recently, leprosy was the most common cause of neuropathy in the world. Hepatitis C can lead to the production of antibodies called *cryoglobulins,* which go on to cause neuropathy. Infection with HIV, the cause of acquired immunodeficiency syndrome (AIDS), can cause neuropathy. Although the virus does not infect neurons directly, it does infect cells that support the health of neurons and their axons.

Neuropathy caused by diphtheria is caused by a toxin produced by the bacterium *Corynebacterium diphtheriae*. The toxin damages myelin, resulting in a demyelinating neuropathy.

As discussed in chapter 2, Guillain-Barré syndrome is a postinfectious autoimmune neuropathy. Antibodies produced against an infection with any number of viruses or bacteria can cause demyelinating neuropathy. Infection with a bacterium called *Campylobacter jejuni*, which causes a diarrheal illness, leads to axonal neuropathy as a result of an autoimmune mechanism. This is called *acute axonal neuropathy*. Postinfectious neuropathy often progresses quickly, over days to weeks, and this progression will alert your doctor to consider this cause of neuropathy.

Neuropathy Associated with Medication

Many medications can cause neuropathy. Sometimes the nerve damage is a common, almost expected, side effect, and other times it is rare. Medications that can cause neuropathy do not necessarily cause neuropathy in all people who take them. Predicting who will develop neuropathy with a given medication is typically not possible, though people who have other risk factors for neuropathy may be more likely to have this side effect. Symptoms may appear soon after a medication is started or may not begin for many months. Medication damages nerves through any of several mechanisms: for example, the drug may interfere with a specific aspect of cellular metabolism or with production of energy-containing molecules. Medication can also interfere with the transport of energy-containing molecules and structural building materials between the cell body and the axon. Damage to the cells that produce myelin is another possible mechanism. Table 4.2 lists the medications that may be problematic. Please note that any list of medications expands as new medications are approved for use; therefore, this table is not comprehensive.

With some medications, particularly drugs used to treat cancer or HIV infection, neuropathy is an expected side effect, which can limit use of the medication. Most neuropathies caused by medication are length-dependent axonal neuropathies. Rarely, medication causes damage to the myelin. If you notice symptoms of neuropathy weeks to months after starting a new medication, talk with your doctor.

Sometimes both the illness and the medication used to treat the illness can cause neuropathy. A careful history of your symptoms should enable your doctor to determine if neuropathic symptoms are due to illness or the medication used to treat the illness.

Symptoms usually improve after the offending medication is stopped, but that may not happen right away. Some medicines are stored in the body, and it takes time for them to be cleared.

Table 4.2 Medications That Can Cause Neuropathy

NAME OF MEDICATION	USED TO TREAT
Amiodarone	Abnormal heart rhythm
Bortezomib	Bone marrow cancer
Carboplatin	Cancer
Chloramphenicol	Serious bacterial infections
Chloroquine	Malaria, autoimmune disorders
Cisplatin	Cancer
Colchicine	Gout
Cytarabine	Cancer
Dapsone	Leprosy, skin diseases
Didanosine	HIV infection
Disulfiram	Alcohol addiction
Docetaxel	Cancer
Etanercept	Rheumatoid arthritis
Ethambutol	Tuberculosis
Fluoroquinolones (class of antibiotics)	Bacterial infections
Gold	Rheumatoid arthritis
Hydralazine	High blood pressure
Hydroxychloroquine	Malaria, autoimmune disorders
Infliximab	Bone marrow cancer
Isoniazid	Tuberculosis
Leflunomide	Rheumatoid arthritis and psoriasis
Lenalidomide	Bone marrow cancer
Metronidazole	Bacterial infections, symptoms of rosacea
Misonidazole	Cancer (used in radiation treatment)
Nitrofurantoin	Urinary tract infection
Oxaliplatin	Cancer
Paclitaxel	Cancer
Phenytoin	Seizures
Procainamide	Abnormal heart rhythm
Procarbazine	Cancer
Pyridoxine (vitamin B6)	Vitamin B6 deficiency (or as a dietary supplement, which can lead to B6 toxicity)
Stavudine	HIV infection
Suramin	Kaposi's sarcoma
Thalidomide	Multiple myeloma, discoid lupus erythematosus
Vinblastine	Cancer
Vincristine	Cancer
Zalcitabine	HIV infection

Sometimes the neuropathy will progress for a while even after the medicine is stopped. In some people, medication-induced neuropathy will resolve completely; in some, only partially; and in a few, not at all. It is not possible to predict what will happen to an individual. For some medications, genetic differences may lead to an increased risk of developing neuropathy. In the future, genetic testing for these variations may be standard to predict a person's risk of developing neuropathy with a certain medication. When your doctor decides on medication, he takes into account the benefits as well as the possible side effects and strikes a balance.

Toxins

Heavy or even regular alcohol use is a common cause of neuropathy. The exact mechanism of alcoholic neuropathy is not known but likely includes direct poisoning of the neuron cell body and the effects of poor nutrition associated with alcoholism. Alcohol is directly toxic to nerves, however, so even in those with a healthy diet, daily use can cause damage. Patients often ask about the heart health benefits of a daily glass or two of red wine. Any possible heart health benefits have to be balanced by the possible side effect of neuropathy. Certainly, I advise those who are already suffering with neuropathy not to "kick their nerves when they are down."

Alcohol is not the only substance that is toxic to nerves. (Table 4.3 lists toxins that can cause neuropathy.) Industrial chemicals such as carbon disulfide and dioxin (alone or as a contaminant of Agent Orange) can cause nerve damage. Exposure to high levels of heavy metals, such as lead, mercury, thallium, or arsenic, can also lead to neuropathy. High-dose or chronic lead exposure causes selective damage to motor axons, resulting in weakness without significant pain or numbness. Exposure to thallium causes a rapidly progressive, painful neuropathy associated with hair loss. Neuropathies from chemicals and heavy metals are usually the result of industrial exposures,

Table 4.3 Toxins That Can Cause Neuropathy

Acrylamide
Arsenic
Brevetoxin (from algae by means of the shellfish that eat it)
Buckthorn berry toxin
Carbon disulfide
Ciguatera toxin (from algae by means of the fish that eat it)
Dioxins
Ethanol
Ethylene glycol (antifreeze)
Hexacarbons (in solvents and glues)
Tetrodotoxin (from puffer fish)
Lead
Mercury (acute exposure to a high dose)
Nitrous oxide (causing depletion of vitamin B12)
Organophosphates (insecticide)
Saxitoxin (from algae by means of the shellfish that eat it)
Thallium (associated with hair loss)
Zinc toxicity (leading to copper deficiency)

---

not dental fillings or routine environmental exposures. Organophosphate insecticide can cause neuropathy, but this is seen in large accidental exposures.

Neuropathy Associated with Cancer

Very rarely, cancer itself, as opposed to medications used in the treatment of cancer, can cause neuropathy. This is called *paraneoplastic neuropathy*. Antibodies that are made by the body to attack the cancer sometimes also attack the axon or the myelin coating. These neuropathies are often painful and progress rapidly over weeks to months. This unusual progression may alert your doctor to look for cancer.

Radiation treatment can cause damage to nerves. This damage is focal, meaning it affects only nerves in the field of radiation. The symptoms are similar to that of generalized neuropathy: pain, tingling, numbness, and weakness. Symptoms can start at the time of treatment or many months to years after treatment. If you have had radiation treatment in the past, it is important to tell your doctor because this may explain symptoms of neuropathy that are in only one area of your body.

Damage to the Blood Supply

Like all tissues in the body, nerves require a blood supply. Tiny arteries bring blood to the neuron cell body, nerves, the cells that make myelin, and other supporting cells. Loss of the blood supply will damage nerves. Typical causes include the inflammation of blood vessels associated with autoimmune disease, diabetes-related blockage of the arteries, or constriction of the arteries as a result of cigarette smoking. With each puff of a cigarette, the nicotine that is inhaled causes blood vessels all over the body to constrict, decreasing the amount of blood getting to all tissues, nerves included.

Sometimes, despite testing, the cause of a person's neuropathy is not found. When this happens, the usual course is to treat the symptoms and repeat testing after six months to a year.

CHAPTER 5

How Is Neuropathy Diagnosed?

Listen to your patient: he is telling you the diagnosis.
William Osler, MD (1849–1919), called
the Father of Modern Medicine

As with any medical problem, diagnosing neuropathy requires a medical history, physical examination, and tests. Your
primary care doctor may refer you to a specialist, such as a neurologist or a physiatrist (a rehabilitation medicine doctor). To
make the most of a visit with the doctor, bring a list of the medications you are taking; a list of any allergies, including what
happens to you during an allergic reaction; the office note from
other medical visits; and the results of any tests, including a
compact disc of any scans you have had. If possible, take with
you a written timeline of when symptoms occurred. Write out
a list of questions you want to ask the doctor. Preparing for the
visit will make the visit more effective and help you avoid for-
getting important information and questions.

Medical History

This part of the process is particularly important in the diagnosis of neuropathy and its cause because most neuropathies
have similar symptoms and show similar findings on examination. By talking with you, the doctor arrives at the initial diagnosis and has clues about what's causing your symptoms.

What doctors call "history of the present illness" is the story of symptoms that brings a person to the doctor. This story can evolve over many years or just a few hours. Doctors are creatures of their training, and we are trained to listen to the story in chronological order, so the first question we often ask is "When did you first notice something?" Although it is tempting to ask the doctor to just read the office notes you bring, it is more helpful to the doctor to hear the story, as it unfolded, from you. She will want to know how long symptoms have been occurring; if anything in particular was happening at the time the symptoms began; if they have gotten better, worse, or stayed the same since they started; and, most importantly, what these symptoms mean to you.

This part of the office visit should be the longest. The doctor will want to know about your entire medical history. The long forms and endless questions can be trying, particularly for someone in pain, but they are meaningful for the physician and useful to you. Information about past medical problems as well as current and past medications is essential to provide because neuropathy may be related to these. Prior surgeries, particularly those for pinched nerves in the spine, are important for the doctor to know about, as those conditions can influence your symptoms and examination. Family history is significant, because some neuropathies and illnesses that can lead to neuropathy are inherited. An updated list of allergies to medication is critical information when the physician is deciding on treatment. The doctor will want to know if you drink alcohol (and how much), smoke, or use recreational drugs, because these activities can cause or aggravate the symptoms of neuropathy. Finally, information about your employment and hobbies may give the doctor clues to the cause of your symptoms. Your physician may ask questions that seem odd or overly personal, but your answer to each supplies information that leads to a diagnosis. Remember, whatever you tell the doctor is confidential, and the doctor has heard it all!

The doctor will ask you to describe your symptoms—what they are and where they are. She may ask specifically if you experience numbness, burning, tingling, squeezing, weakness, or feelings of being off balance. The doctor will ask how your symptoms evolved over time. Be prepared to describe any difficulties you have with everyday activities as well as interference with sleep as a result of your symptoms.

The doctor will ask about symptoms related to the autonomic nervous system, such as lightheadedness when standing, dry eyes and mouth, problems with vision, fullness after a small meal, diarrhea and constipation, trouble with bladder function, and presence of sexual dysfunction, including erectile dysfunction if applicable.

The Neurological Examination Decoded

The neurological exam is strange and unlike other examinations. You are asked to do things for the doctor that may seem odd. Why is the doctor examining you in this way, and what is she thinking?

In this section, I go through each part of the exam: mental status, cranial nerves, strength, sensation, reflexes, coordination and balance, and walking, as well as aspects of the general exam that are particularly pertinent to neuropathy, such as inspection of the feet and maneuvers to examine the autonomic system.

Typically, the exam will start with the usual—the doctor or the medical assistant will take your vital signs, including height, weight, pulse, and blood pressure. Blood pressure and pulse may be measured a few times, with you lying down, sitting, and standing. Then the doctor will examine your lungs, heart, blood vessels in the neck, and any other part of your body that may be related to your problem. When performing the neurological examination, the doctor may not perform tasks in the order listed below, but she is thinking in this order. From the neurologist's point of view, the different parts of the exam represent different structures in the nervous system. What she finds on exam serves as a proxy for the function of these structures. So while examining the *outside* of you, the doctor is thinking about the *inside* of you.

Examination of Mental Status

During this part of the exam, the neurologist seeks answers to questions such as these: Is the patient alert and thinking clearly enough to be able to cooperate with the rest of the exam? Are speech, language, and memory intact? Is the person's emotional state appropriate for the situation? You may be asked to recite the date, list your home address, or name the current president. You may be given three words and asked to remember them for later. You may be asked to read a passage, write a sentence, or draw a clock. Each exercise assesses the function of a different part of the brain. For example, damage to the left side of the brain may interfere with the ability to speak or to understand language, and damage to the right side of the brain may interfere with spatial processing, such as the ability to copy a three-dimensional drawing or an arrangement of blocks.

Examination of the Cranial Nerves

Cranial nerves are the nerves of the face and head. The doctor will shine a light in your eyes to examine whether your pupils constrict appropriately. With autonomic neuropathy, pupils will not constrict to light. She will look into the back of your eyes with an ophthalmoscope to examine the optic nerve, the nerve that runs from the eye into the brain. The neurologist will note movement of your eyes and face. Your senses of taste and smell may be tested. In someone with neuropathy, these senses may be abnormal. The doctor will ask you to "stick out your tongue and say ah." She is looking to see that your tongue and palate move normally.

Examination of Muscle Strength: The Motor Exam

This test is done to measure muscle strength. The doctor will have you contract many different muscles against resistance and grade that strength. Most neurologists use a scale of 0 to 5, where 5 is normal strength, and 0 means the muscle does not move at all. The doctor is thinking not only about whether muscles are weak but also about the *pattern* of weakness. For example, is the weakness symmetrical and in muscles innervated by the longest nerves, like those in the feet and lower legs? This pattern is consistent with an axonal, length-dependent, dying-back neuropathy. If the pattern of weakness is different from this, the doctor will be thinking about other possible explanations for your symptoms. For example, is the weakness in muscles closest to the trunk? This suggests a demyelinating neuropathy or a primary problem with the muscles. Is the weakness in muscles that receive their nerve supply from only one nerve or one level of the spinal cord? This suggests damage to one nerve or one nerve root as it exits the spine, not a generalized disorder of nerves. Is the weakness on only one side of the body? This is more in keeping with a problem in the brain or spinal cord.

The doctor will also look at the muscles to see if they are the correct size. With neuropathy, muscle atrophy may be visible. The muscles are examined for twitches, called *fasciculations*, which can be a sign that the nerve or motor neurons are damaged. The doctor will also examine tone. This is the resistance felt to passive movement of a limb. If the tone is abnormally increased, the problem is in the brain or spinal cord, not in the nerves.

Examination of Sensation

The doctor will test different sensations that correspond to the different axon sizes. The sensory exam is particularly sensitive to the length-dependent pattern of axonal neuropathy. Loss of sensation will first be noticed in the feet, slowly moving up the legs over time to eventually extend to the hands and arms.

To test small-axon modalities, such as pain and temperature, the neurologist may lightly poke the skin with a one-use-only pin and place a cold metal tuning fork or test tube filled with water on the skin. If there is sensory loss in the feet, she will be looking to see how high up in the leg the sensory loss extends, and whether it goes up into the hands as well. You may be asked to quantify the loss. When I perform this test, I put a cold tuning fork on a patch of skin that has normal sensation and then on an area of decreased sensation and ask, "If this degree of cold is worth a dollar (normal area), how much is this worth (area of decrease)?"

Large-axon modalities, such as vibration and joint position sense, will be tested. The doctor will apply a vibrating 128 Hz tuning fork to your big toe and ask if you can feel it. If you cannot feel it on your toe, she will move the tuning fork up to the ankle, knee, and hip. To test joint position sense, the doctor will have you close your eyes and will move your big toe or thumb up or down and ask you the direction of movement. This can also be tested by having you stand with your eyes closed, feet close together, and hands stretched out in front. The ability to keep your balance in this position is a measure of how well joint position sense from your toes, ankles, and knees is being conveyed to your brain. This test is called the Romberg maneuver, named after Moritz Romberg, the doctor who invented it.

Examination of Tendon Reflexes

The neurologist taps on your knee with a hammer, and your leg kicks out. What is the doctor doing and why? A medical hammer is used to tap on a muscle tendon. A tendon is the connective tissue that attaches a muscle to a bone. Tapping on the tendon quickly stretches the muscle a little bit. This feeling of stretch is detected by specialized muscle cells and then transmitted along a sensory nerve from those muscle cells to the spinal cord, which, through a reflex, causes the muscle to contract. The doctor is tapping on the tendon of the quadriceps muscle (the muscle on the front of the thigh) that runs over the knee joint.

When that muscle contracts, it extends your knee. In neuropathy, reflexes are often diminished or absent because the nerve that brings the information about the muscle stretch to the spinal cord is damaged and can't transmit the message. Commonly tested reflexes include those at the ankle, knee, wrist, and elbow. In neuropathy, the ankle reflex is often diminished or absent because it depends on the longest nerves. In severe neuropathy, all reflexes may be absent. Reflexes that are too brisk suggest a problem in the spinal cord or brain rather than in the nerve.

Examination of Coordination and Walking

These are tests of the largest axons, those that mediate joint position sense, as well as the cerebellum, the little brain, which hangs off the back of the brain and regulates coordination. The doctor may ask you to take your index finger and touch your nose and then the examiner's finger, and then take one heel and run it down the shin of the other leg. She will ask you to walk normally and then to walk with one foot in front of the other, as if on a tightrope.

Examination of Autonomic Function

Testing of autonomic function is scattered throughout the exam. These parts of the exam evaluate function of autonomic nerves:

- Shining a light into your eyes to see if your pupils constrict properly
- Taking your blood pressure while you are in different positions—lying down, sitting, and standing—to look for a drop in blood pressure

- Taking your pulse and asking you to take deep breaths (Normally, the heart rate increases when you breathe in and slows when you exhale. This is mediated by autonomic nerves.)

Examination of the Feet

For people with neuropathy, this may be one of the most important parts of the exam. The doctor will look for cuts, blisters, signs of infection, and deformities of the foot that occur with muscle weakness and lack of sensation.

At the End of the Office Visit, What Is the Doctor Thinking?

In the office, I ask my patients: "Do you want to know what I'm thinking?" While the patient is getting dressed, I take a moment to think about what I have heard and seen on the exam. Is this truly a peripheral neuropathy or something else? Is the cause something common and obvious, or does it remain unknown? What tests would be useful? Is treatment necessary now, and if it is, what sort of treatment is best? Doctors should not be keeping these thoughts to themselves! During your office visit, the doctor should talk with you about what she is thinking.

CHAPTER 6

Tests

Early testing and diagnosis helped me to gain control of my situation and work proactively with my doctors. The tests performed on me have ranged from uncomfortable to surprisingly simple, but the doctors have always explained the need for each test. Jimmy Dean said: "I can't change the direction of the wind, but I can adjust my sails to always reach my destination." It is how you approach life's challenges that makes the difference in how you proceed!

Going to the doctor means getting tests. The tests are used not only to diagnose neuropathy and its cause but to rule out other possible causes for your symptoms and exam abnormalities. There are many types of tests, including blood and urine tests, electrical testing of nerves and muscles, biopsies, imaging studies, and special tests of autonomic function. Not all people with neuropathy receive all of these tests. Your doctor will order some of the tests based on your medical history and examination. The American Academy of Neurology has published guidelines for patients regarding evaluation of neuropathy (aka distal symmetric polyneuropathy, or neuritis). Those guidelines can be found at www.aan.com/Guidelines/Home/GetGuideline Content/323.

Don't be shy about asking your doctor what each test entails and what he is looking for with each test. Ask about the procedure and the possible risks and side effects. If one test sounds too risky or uncomfortable to you, ask if another test can give the same information. As a patient you are entitled to a copy of your test results and an explanation of these results. If the doctor is not providing satisfactory answers, ask again. If you feel that the doctor is not partnering with you in developing an evaluation and treatment plan, it is fine to get a second opinion or find a different doctor.

Blood Tests

Blood will be drawn from a vein to look for common causes of neuropathy, such as diabetes; dysfunction of the kidney, thyroid, or bone marrow; and some vitamin deficiencies or toxicities. Blood testing is safe, and adverse effects, including bleeding, bruising, and infection, are very uncommon. The following sections describe common blood tests.

Complete Blood Count

Red blood cells carry oxygen in the blood to organs, while white blood cells fight infection. The complete blood count measures the number of red and white blood cells and the percentage of each type of white blood cell. There is only one type of red blood cell. If the number of cells is not normal, this result could point to a problem in the bone marrow, where red and white cells are produced. Some bone marrow cancers can cause neuropathy by producing antibodies that cross-react with proteins on nerves or by producing too much antibody that can deposit in tissues and nerves as an insoluble substance called amyloid. In addition, the size of the red blood cells can give a clue to other problems. For example, red blood cells that are too large are seen in people who have vitamin B12 deficiency.

Vitamin Levels

Lack of vitamins B1 or B12 and too much vitamin B6 can cause neuropathy. Vitamin B12 is involved in the production of myelin. A lack of B12 can lead to abnormal myelin production and neuropathy. Too high a level of vitamin B6 is toxic to sensory neurons.

Thyroid Hormone

Underactive thyroid function can cause neuropathy. Although this is a rare cause of neuropathy, it is easily treatable, and your doctor would not want to miss it.

Blood Urea Nitrogen and Creatinine

Blood urea nitrogen and creatinine levels are measures of kidney function. The kidney filters out creatinine, urea, and other chemicals that are byproducts of normal metabolism. If kidneys are not working normally, creatinine and urea will build up in the blood. Kidney disease, over time, can cause neuropathy because of incomplete filtration of toxins from the blood.

Tests for Diabetes Mellitus

Diabetes mellitus is the most common cause of neuropathy in the world. The word *diabetes* comes from Greek, meaning "to flow," and *mellitus* means "like honey." Diabetes mellitus is to flow sweet. This name comes from the diagnostic test that was done many years ago, when laboratory technicians tasted urine samples for sweetness. Sugar from the blood overflows into the urine and makes it taste sweet.

Fasting Blood Sugar (Glucose) Level
You will be asked to have your blood drawn in the morning, before you eat. High levels of blood sugar (glucose) are a clue to the diagnosis of diabetes.

Hemoglobin A1c

Hemoglobin is an iron-containing molecule in red blood cells that carries oxygen. Sugar in the blood can attach to hemoglobin. The hemoglobin A1c test measures the percentage of hemoglobin that has sugar attached to it. A red blood cell lasts in the circulation for about ten days, so the results of this test show blood sugar levels over the past week or so. A number of 6.1 to 6.5 percent (depending on the testing lab) or more is suspicious for diabetes.

Two-Hour Glucose Tolerance Test

Even if the level of glucose in your blood is normal when fasting, you may not be metabolizing glucose quickly enough after you eat. For the two-hour glucose tolerance test, after your blood sugar is tested, you drink a small amount of a very sweet liquid. Your blood sugar will be tested one hour and then two hours after you finish the drink. Normally, blood sugar will go up and then come down during this time. If your blood sugar stays high, that is a clue to the presence of diabetes.

Rapid Plasma Reagin

Rapid plasma reagin (RPR) is a test for syphilis. Syphilis does not cause neuropathy but can cause something that could be mistaken for neuropathy. This is a routine test and does not mean that your doctor thinks you have syphilis.

Test for Human Immunodeficiency Virus

This test looks for antibodies made to attack the virus. It can take up to six months after exposure to develop antibodies to HIV.

Test for Hepatitis C

Hepatitis alone rarely causes neuropathy. Hepatitis C can be associated with the production of cryoglobulins in the blood. These are proteins that precipitate (separate) from the blood in a test tube when the blood is chilled. Blood tests can be done looking for antibodies to hepatitis C as well as looking for cryoglobulins directly.

Tests for Lyme Disease

Lyme disease does not cause a true neuropathy, but it can cause other problems that look like neuropathy. Testing for Lyme disease is not as straightforward as testing for other infections. More than one test must be positive. Usually, a screening test called ELISA is done, and if this is positive, a more specific test, called a Western blot, is done. In addition, pieces of the Lyme disease bacteria can also be detected.

Serum Protein Electrophoresis and Immunofixation

Serum protein electrophoresis and immunofixation is a long name for two tests that are done together to look for abnormal proteins in the blood made by cells in the bone marrow. These proteins may be antibodies that can attach to nerves and damage them. Sometimes the proteins point to cancer of the bone marrow, and sometimes they are benign.

Tests of Liver Function

Liver function tests look for enzymes that are released by liver cells when they are damaged. The enzyme levels give an overall view of the liver's function, which can be affected in many illnesses that also cause neuropathy. Elevation of liver enzymes may signal an infection, such as hepatitis, or damage from alcohol use.

Erythrocyte Sedimentation Rate

Erythrocyte is another name for a red blood cell. The erythrocyte sedimentation rate (ESR) test examines how quickly red blood cells fall to the bottom of a test tube filled with blood. This fall rate is a measure of inflammation throughout the body. A rate that is too fast signals inflammation in the body that can be associated with any of several different diseases.

Less Common Blood Tests

Less common blood tests may be ordered depending on the results of the routine tests and on your personal medical history. Some of these less common tests are briefly described below.

Screen for Heavy Metals

Long-term exposure to metals such as lead, mercury, and arsenic can cause nerve damage. Usually when this screen is ordered, the person has a well-known exposure through a job or hobby. This test should be done on blood or urine, not on hair from your head. Testing done on hair is contaminated by exposure to air pollution. Unscrupulous testing facilities test hair for contaminants and produce alarming reports.

Tests for Autoimmune Connective Tissue Diseases

Sometimes the body produces antibodies against itself, and these can be measured in the blood. Autoimmune diseases may be associated with neuropathy, including systemic lupus erythematosus, Sjögren's disease, and many others.

Tests for Porphyria

Porphyria is a rare genetic disease in which the body produces abnormal hemoglobin. People may feel fine until the use of certain medications brings out symptoms. Neuropathy due to porphyria is demyelinating and comes on quickly. It may be associated with abdominal pain, vomiting, and depressed mental state. This test measures the level of a certain enzyme in red blood cells.

Testing for Inherited Causes of Neuropathy

Neuropathy can be inherited in two general ways. One way is to inherit a gene that causes neuropathy. The other is to inherit a disease that has neuropathy as a symptom. Many inherited genetic mutations can directly lead to neuropathy. Inherited neuropathies may represent a larger proportion of neuropathies than previously thought. For some of these disorders, commercial or research lab testing is available. The list of genetic tests is increasing rapidly, and if your doctor suspects an inherited neuropathy, then a current search for a possible blood test is in order. The most common directly inherited neuropathy is called Charcot-Marie-Tooth disease type 1. It is named after the three physicians who first described it over one hundred years ago. This neuropathy is inherited in an autosomal dominant fashion, meaning that having only one copy of the mutated gene is enough to get the disease. For each gene, you have two copies, one from your mother and one from your father. With Charcot-Marie-Tooth disease, usually one parent has also had symptoms. Each child of that parent has a 50 percent chance of getting the mutated gene, and hence the neuropathy. Other neuropathies show an autosomal recessive pattern, meaning that you need to inherit two copies of the mutated gene for the disease to occur. An X-linked pattern means that the disease affects only males, who have one X chromosome and one Y chromosome (while females have two X's). In these forms of inheritance, a family history may not be obvious. Your doctor will determine which genetic tests are appropriate.

Some illnesses that are inherited and have neuropathy as a symptom include Pompe disease (involving a metabolic error), familial amyloidosis (in which an abnormal protein is made and deposited along nerves), and Friedreich's ataxia (in which there is a deficiency in a cellular protein).

I am sometimes asked if the results of genetic testing can

be used to deprive a person of insurance. A full discussion is outside the scope of this book, but the federal Genetic Information Nondiscrimination Act of 2008 protects people from discrimination by health insurers and employers on the basis of genetic testing results. This law does not apply, however, to life, disability, and long-term care insurers.

Urine Tests

Your doctor may ask for a urine sample, either a one-time sample or a collection over twenty-four hours. If you are asked to collect a twenty-four-hour sample, your doctor will give you a container for holding the urine. The kidney makes urine by filtering blood, then reabsorbing important nutrients and electrolytes back into the blood. What is left over is urine. There should be no sugar or protein in the urine. The presence of sugar points to diabetes, with sugar overflowing from the blood to the urine. The presence of protein points to kidney dysfunction.

Electrocardiogram

If you experience lightheadedness or fainting, your doctor may order an electrocardiogram (ECG) to make sure your heart rate (the number of times per minute your heart beats) and rhythm are normal. An ECG measures the electrical activity produced by the heart. In this test sticky rubber patches (called *leads*) are attached to the chest wall, with wires that run from these patches to the ECG machine. If hair interferes with the leads sticking, some patches of skin may be shaved. The test takes about fifteen minutes to perform, and the patches are then removed. There are no side effects from this test.

Nerve Conduction Studies and Electromyography

Nerve conduction studies and electromyography (NCS/EMG) is a two-part electrical test of the function of nerves and muscles. The purpose of the test is to determine whether any nerves are malfunctioning, and if so, to identify the type of problem (axonal versus myelin), the severity of the problem, and the pattern of nerves and muscles that are abnormal. An EMG machine is a computer that detects and analyzes the electrical activity produced by nerves and muscles.

As discussed in chapter 1, nerves are like wires in many ways, including how they conduct electricity. For the NCS portion of the test, the doctor or a technician will tape some metal or plastic electrodes over a muscle or a patch of skin, then apply a small amount of electricity to stimulate the nerve that goes to that muscle or patch of skin. The electrodes on the skin are recording the electrical activity of the stimulated nerve or muscle. With each stimulation, you may feel your muscles contract a little bit. Several parameters are recorded, including the size and speed of the response. During the EMG portion of the test, the skin covering a muscle is cleansed with alcohol, and then a very thin, sterile, one-use needlelike electrode is inserted through the skin and into the muscle. You will be asked to contract and relax the muscle. No electricity goes through the needle; it is a recording device. There may be a very small amount of blood from the needle prick. During this part of the test, you will see waves running across the EMG screen and hear noise coming from the machine—the doctor is looking at and listening to the electricity generated by the muscle membrane when the muscle contracts. In preparation for the test, you will be asked to bathe the day of the test to get rid of oil on the skin and to refrain from using moisturizer, which would interfere with securing electrodes to the skin.

These procedures may sound painful; different people react differently to the test, but in the right hands, it should be merely uncomfortable. The amount of electricity and the number of shocks used should be the minimum needed to give the necessary information, and the needle electrode is quite thin. People ask about the use of a local anesthetic. That would help relieve discomfort of the skin, but it is not possible to numb the muscle. Some doctors apply a local anesthetic spray or cream before the test. Ask the doctor if he will apply a local anesthetic.

Before the test, the doctor will ask if you are taking blood thinners and will examine your skin to make sure there are no infections. Using a blood thinner does not preclude the needle exam, but the doctor will want to know the results of a blood test to make sure your blood is not too thinned. Normally, the EMG portion does not cause bleeding because the electrode is solid (not hollow like a needle) and ultrathin. Infection is extremely rare because each needle is sterile, disposable, and used only for one person. The nerve conduction portion does not leave any marks, although the doctor will use a pen to mark the spot where he stimulated the nerve. Stimulating the nerves with electricity in this test does not damage them because very little electricity is used. Sometimes people are a little sore after the test. Applying ice over the skin and muscles tested can relieve the discomfort.

One disadvantage of this test is that it has trouble detecting neuropathy that affects only the thinnest axons, like those mediating pain and autonomic function. Other tests, such as autonomic testing, quantitative sensory testing, and skin and nerve biopsy are better at detecting this sort of neuropathy.

Quantitative Sensory Testing

Quantitative sensory testing (QST) is a specialized test that examines thin, medium, and thick axons. The QST is more sensitive than nerve conduction studies in looking for damage to the thinnest axons. This test is used in clinical research trials more than in regular practice because it requires a special machine and a technician trained in its use. In preparation for the QST, you will be asked to bathe the day of the test to get rid of oil on the skin and to refrain from using moisturizer, which would interfere with sensation on the skin as well as with securing the instrument. If there is excessive hair over the area to be tested, the technician may shave that area before the test.

Sensory modalities that are typically tested include heat that is felt as pain as well as sensitivity to light touch and vibration. In the test, a small patch of skin over the top of the foot is examined to determine the lowest threshold for detection of touch, vibration, and heat that feels like pain.

Testing of heat that feels like pain sounds a lot worse than it is. In this portion of the test, a small ceramic cube is taped to the top of the foot. The cube slowly heats up, and you are asked to press a button as soon as the heat feels like pain. When you press the button, the heating stops. The pain sensation is minimal because you are asked to press the stop button as soon as you feel a change from heat to pain. The amount of heat applied is limited, so that even if you do not feel the heat at all, there is no risk of skin or nerve damage.

The test for touch sensation involves using a series of nylon filaments that range in diameter from extremely thin to quite thick. You close your eyes or wear an eye mask, and the examiner touches your big toe with filaments of different diameters. It is more difficult to feel the thinnest filaments than it is to feel the thickest. The technician will record the thinnest filament diameter that you can feel.

For testing of vibration sensation, you sit in a chair in a quiet room. A small tuning fork that is attached by a cable to the QST machine is placed on top of your foot. The amount of vibration is regulated by the machine. It starts off with a small amount and slowly increases to a larger degree of vibration. As soon as you feel vibration, you press a button. The minimum level of vibration that you can detect is recorded.

Each test is repeated several times to get a measure of the best response, and so the QST requires prolonged cooperation and concentration on the tasks. There are no side effects from the test.

Ultrasound

In ultrasound, sound waves are sent to a structure inside the body. The waves bounce off and return to a detector that makes a picture from those returning sound waves. People are most familiar with ultrasound for looking at babies before they are born, but ultrasound is gaining in popularity for evaluating nerves and muscles. During this test, a handheld plastic probe is coated with gel and then pressed lightly over the muscle or nerve to be viewed. Ultrasound waves are emitted from the probe, and the resulting picture is displayed on a screen. Ultrasound waves are not harmful. There are no complications or side effects from the test, and it is tolerated well. The gel is water soluble and is wiped off when the test is finished.

Tests of Autonomic Function

Tests of autonomic function are useful to evaluate small-axon function. They are not commonly obtained, however, because they require specialized equipment and technician training. Your doctor may feel that the history you relate is enough to conclude that this part of the nervous system is involved in your symptoms.

Tilt Table Test

This is test of blood pressure and heart rate. You lie flat on a table, and your blood pressure and heart rate are measured. The table slowly tilts up, raising your head and lowering your feet, and your blood pressure and heart rate are again measured. Normally, as the head is raised, blood pressure and heart rate increase to keep blood pumping against gravity, up toward the head. This compensation mechanism is mediated by autonomic nerves. If the nerves are damaged, your heart rate and blood pressure will not increase, and you may feel lightheaded. The testing takes about thirty minutes. It is generally well tolerated.

Possible adverse effects include lightheadedness, fainting, and a feeling of nausea.

Quantitative Sudomotor Axon Reflex Test (QSART)

Sudomotor refers to the autonomic nerves that supply sweat glands. The quantitative sudomotor axon reflex test (QSART) can be performed in many ways. In the most common, a mild electrical shock is given to the palm of the hand, and surface electrodes stuck to the palm record the amount of sweat produced. This amount is displayed as a curved line on a screen. Normally, the electrical shock makes the palm sweat. If the autonomic nerves are damaged, sweating will be decreased or absent. Although the electrical shock is uncomfortable, it is not painful, and there are no adverse side effects of the test.

Heart Rate Deep Breathing

When you take a deep breath, your heart rate increases, and when you exhale, it decreases. When you inhale, your rib cage moves outward and creates a small vacuum, drawing air into the lungs. This is like a bellows used to stoke a fire. The decreased pressure in the chest cavity draws more blood from the body to the heart. The heart has to pump faster to deal with the increased amount of blood. When you exhale, the opposite occurs—the pressure in your chest increases, decreasing the amount of blood returning to your heart and therefore slowing your heart rate. These responses are mediated by autonomic nerves. When these nerves are damaged, the heart rate stays the same during inhalation and exhalation. In this test, an electrode is placed on the finger to measure the heart rate, and a belt is fastened around the waist to measure breathing. The results are displayed as two waves on a computer screen. The test is not uncomfortable, although you are asked to take very deep breaths. Sometimes people become lightheaded while taking deep breaths, but there are usually no adverse effects from the test.

Tests of Bladder Function

If you are having difficulty urinating or are having recurrent bladder infections, you may be referred to a urologist for examination and specialized tests of bladder function. The urologist will ask about other medications you are taking because many different types of medicine can inhibit bladder contraction. There are many tests of bladder function, but the simplest is called a *postvoid residual*. In this test you will be asked to empty your bladder as completely as possible. After that, an ultrasound of the bladder is performed to measure the amount of urine left in the bladder. Alternatively, a thin rubber tube, called a *catheter*, may be placed in the bladder to drain it and measure the amount of urine.

Computerized Axial Tomography and Magnetic Resonance Imaging

CT scans and MRIs are two ways to look at the brain and spinal cord. If your doctor thinks that your symptoms may be related to a pinched nerve in the back or a problem in the spinal cord or brain, one of these tests may be ordered. An MRI uses a magnet to make the picture, and a CT scan uses radiation. MRI is better at seeing soft tissue, such as the spinal cord and nerve roots. A CT scan is better at seeing blood and bone. Those with implanted medical devices, such as pacemakers and some metal implants, cannot have an MRI because of safety concerns related to the magnet.

For both tests, you are asked to lie on your back on a narrow table. Bolsters can be placed under the knees for comfort. The table moves into the machine, which is shaped like a big doughnut. The MRI machine may produce a mild clanging sound. You will be able to speak with the technician during the test. Sometimes the studies are ordered with contrast. Contrast is a solution that is drunk or injected into a vein before the scan to highlight certain abnormalities.

Before the test, your doctor or the technician will ask if you have an allergy to shellfish, because that allergy may produce an allergic reaction to CT contrast. People who have diabetes and reduced kidney function are at risk for kidney damage caused by the CT or MRI contrast. Before the test, your doctor will ask if you have diabetes and will get blood tests to look at kidney function in order to avoid this complication. The tests usually last twenty to thirty minutes. Both are usually well tolerated. The CT scan involves exposure to radiation, but usually only one scan is needed. Those who are claustrophobic may find these scans uncomfortable. Open scanners are becoming available. An eye mask can make the test easier to tolerate, and some people do well with a small dose of sedative before the test.

Biopsies

A biopsy is a procedure in which a small piece of tissue is removed and examined under a microscope. Two types of biopsies are sometimes used in the diagnosis of neuropathy.

Skin Biopsy

Skin biopsy is a technique for diagnosing small-axon neuropathy. After you receive local anesthetic, the doctor will remove a small, shallow core of skin from your thigh and another from just above your ankle. The skin is stained, and the number of very small axons is counted. This number is compared to that of normal age-matched samples. If the density of small axons is less than it should be, that is a clue to the presence of a small-axon neuropathy. Since axonal neuropathies are typically length dependent, the skin from the ankle will have fewer axons than the skin from the thigh, where nerves are shorter.

Skin biopsy can also give an indirect measure of autonomic neuropathy. Sweat glands in the skin are innervated by autonomic nerves, and sweat gland innervation can be evaluated in the biopsy. The procedure is bloodless, and side effects are rare. A small scar might remain at the site of the biopsy. Those with diabetes or severe neuropathy may have trouble with the surgical wound healing.

Nerve Biopsy

Improvements in blood testing and NCS/EMG have decreased the need for nerve biopsy. Nowadays, one common reason for a nerve biopsy is to look for something infiltrating the nerves, such as cancer cells or abnormal proteins. Another is to look for vasculitis, which is inflammation of the blood vessels that nourish the nerves. For both diagnoses, it is important to have a *tissue diagnosis*, proof of the problem in a tissue sample, because both sorts of problems require treatment that may have serious side effects. The most common nerve to be biopsied is the sural nerve. This nerve contains only sensory axons and runs from the leg to the outside of the ankle into the foot. Using local anesthesia, a surgeon removes a piece of nerve about an inch long from behind your ankle. The nerve is sent to the pathology laboratory, where it is preserved, cut into extremely thin slices, stained, and evaluated under the microscope by a pathologist. This procedure is typically well tolerated but does leave a patch of numbness on the side of the foot. The nerve does not grow back because the surgery leaves scar tissue at the end of the nerve. Rarely, nerve biopsy may lead to what is called *anesthesia dolorosa*, meaning numbness and pain, where the patch of numb skin is also painful. If this occurs, it usually slowly resolves over months.

Lumbar Puncture (Spinal Tap)

Occasionally, your doctor may want to perform a lumbar puncture, also called a spinal tap. This test is done to obtain a sample of the fluid that surrounds and bathes the brain and spinal cord. The fluid is called *cerebrospinal fluid*. Lumbar puncture is done to look for a more unusual type of neuropathy called demyelinating neuropathy, which occurs when the myelin coating around the nerves is damaged. Certain proteins are released from myelin into the fluid, and they can be measured. Informed consent from you is required before the procedure. How the test is performed, the reason for the test, the risks of not having the test, and the possible side effects will be explained. Lumbar puncture is done under sterile conditions at the bedside. A small patch of skin over the lower back is cleaned with antibacterial solution, and then local anesthetic is injected under the skin in the center of the back. After this, a thin, sterile needle is placed between two backbones, puncturing the sac that contains the fluid. About a tablespoon of fluid is removed. It replenishes itself in a few hours. The fluid is tested for protein, sugar, red and white blood cells, infectious agents, and other chemicals.

The procedure is routine, and complications are rare. Occasionally, the needle enters a vein, causing blood to come out of the needle. In those instances, pressure is put on the site for a few minutes, and the needle is moved to another level of the back. Infection is a possible complication but is rare because the procedure is done under sterile conditions with a sterile, one-use-only needle. Even more rarely, the needle brushes up against a nerve root, causing pain that radiates down one leg. If this occurs, the procedure is stopped, and the needle is adjusted. This usually does not cause damage to the nerve root.

After the procedure, some people have a headache that is worse when sitting up and better when lying down. This headache is thought to be the result of lower pressure in the spinal column after fluid is removed or a small leak of cerebrospinal fluid. When a headache occurs, treatment starts with conservative measures, such as bed rest and drinking fluids that contain caffeine. The caffeine causes blood vessels to constrict and indirectly raises the cerebrospinal fluid pressure. If the headache continues for more than a few days or is severe, a *blood patch* can be performed. In this procedure, a small amount of blood is drawn from the arm, just like when blood is taken for testing, but this blood is then injected into the area where the lumbar puncture needle had been. The idea is that the blood will clot and block off any small hole that is leaking. This is a very effective treatment. It is usually performed by an anesthesiologist in an emergency room or outpatient facility.

After the Tests: What Is the Doctor Thinking?

After the tests, the doctor is considering whether the medical history, physical examination, and test results support the diagnosis of neuropathy. If so, what type of neuropathy is it, and is there evidence of a probable cause? If not, what else could explain the symptoms and examination findings? Is further testing needed? Sometimes, a diagnosis of neuropathy is made, but the cause remains elusive. The next step may be to treat your symptoms and reevaluate you after time has passed. This is a frustrating outcome for patients but is sometimes the only honest answer your doctor can give.

If testing is complete and a diagnosis is made, the next thing the doctor thinks about is explaining the diagnosis to you, answering your questions and discussing treatment and lifestyle modifications.

CHAPTER 7

Treatment of Neuropathy

Cure sometimes, treat often, comfort always.

Attributed to Hippocrates (460–370 B.C.E.)

~~~~~~

The physician should not treat the disease but the patient who is suffering from it.

Moses Maimonides (1135–1204)

~~~~~~

When talking to patients about treatment, I have found that they are thinking about three different things: treatment of the underlying problem that is causing neuropathy, treatment to make the nerves better, and treatment of symptoms. Unfortunately, no treatments can make the nerves grow back better or faster. They have to do that on their own. In neuropathy, the nerves degenerate from the end back up toward the spinal cord. If the cause of the neuropathy is treated, the nerves can regenerate, but they grow back slowly. Under the best conditions, nerves grow at a rate of one millimeter a day. This translates into one inch each month and one foot each year.

This leaves us with two main categories of treatment: treating the underlying cause of the problem (called *etiologic* treatment) and treating the symptoms (called *symptomatic* treatment). In neuropathy the luxury of the former is rare, and we are often talking about the latter. Etiologic treatment includes controlling blood sugar in diabetes mellitus, eliminating alcohol from the diet, taking vitamin B12 for deficiency, decreasing vitamin B6 if overused, treating thyroid disease, stopping an offending medication (if possible), and so on. For the most common cause of neuropathy, diabetes mellitus, clinical trials have demonstrated that good control of blood sugar is the best treatment. Nerves have a limited ability to heal once they are damaged, so early recognition of diabetes with strict blood sugar control is best.

Sometimes when faced with neuropathy in a patient, a neurologist cannot do much more than give a diagnosis and a probable cause, and then treat the symptoms. What your doctor wants to know is what these symptoms mean to you and what you want to get out of treatment. What do you want made better? That part of the conversation sometimes gets lost. If the doctor does not ask this clearly, it is up to you to tell him what you are looking for in treatment. Being clear about your goals focuses the doctor's treatment plan and helps you get what you need.

Symptomatic treatment falls into three categories: treatment of sensory symptoms, such as pain; treatment of motor symptoms, such as muscle wasting and weakness; and treatment of autonomic symptoms.

Treating Sensory Symptoms

Patients with neuropathy most commonly ask about treatment of unpleasant sensory symptoms. When thinking about treatment, the first question to ask yourself is, Do I need treatment? I approach this by asking patients if the pain and tingling bother them enough that they would want to take medicine every day. If the answer is yes, we talk about which symptoms need to be treated and when. For example, sometimes pain is present twenty-four hours a day; sometimes it is just a problem at night before bed. If the answer is no, then we talk about other sorts of treatment or no treatment at all. Sometimes people can tolerate their symptoms and are interested only in knowing the cause.

As I discuss in chapter 3, doctors think about symptoms as

negative (numbness) or positive (tingling, burning, and pain). No treatment is available for symptoms such as numbness, but many different treatments exist for the symptoms of tingling, burning, and pain. If the only symptom is numbness, treatment is not recommended because none has been proved to help. When treatment of other symptoms is desired, there are many options, some that involve medicine and some that do not.

Neuropathy caused by diabetes is unusual in that changes in diet and close adherence to treatment can slow the progression or reverse the damage of neuropathy. The Diabetes Control and Complications Trial demonstrated that in people who have type 1 diabetes, strict blood sugar control reduces the chance of developing neuropathy by 65 percent after five years. In the study, this effect, to a lesser degree, continued to the fourteen-year mark. Strict control of blood glucose also decreases the risk of eye abnormalities and may decrease the risk of stroke and heart attack associated with diabetes.

Treatment of uncomfortable sensory symptoms is commonly desired. Treatment of pain, tingling, electrical shock–like sensations, and other unpleasant positive symptoms is discussed in the following sections. These symptomatic treatments can be divided into three general categories: treatment without medication, treatment with nonpill medications, and treatment with pills.

Treatment without Medication

You can relieve the pain of neuropathy without medication using various methods. For example, getting a foot rub or using a warm water vibrating foot massager can provide some relief. These techniques work by stimulating axons that mediate deep pressure and vibration, canceling out the input from pain-conducting axons at the level of the spinal cord. These methods are temporary measures, but the effects may last long enough for you to fall asleep.

There is some evidence that electrical stimulation of nerves under the skin (*percutaneous stimulation*) can decrease the pain of neuropathy. In this treatment, low-level electrical stimulation is given via small needles inserted around the painful area. This is done periodically, not continuously. Percutaneous stimulation is not the same as *transcutaneous* electrical nerve stimulation (TENS), in which electrical impulses are applied to the surface of the skin. Although TENS devices are heavily advertised, there is no clear consensus on whether TENS is effective for nerve pain.

Some people get relief with acupuncture, although no scientifically valid studies prove its usefulness in nerve pain. I do not dissuade patients from trying acupuncture as long as they clear the treatment with their primary doctor and seek a reputable practitioner who uses sterile disposable needles to decrease the risk of infection.

Some patients ask me if smoking marijuana is useful for nerve pain. The active ingredients in *Cannabis sativa* include the main psychoactive chemical, a *cannabinoid* called delta-9-tetrohydrocannabinol (delta-9-THC), as well as a nonpsychoactive chemical called *cannabidiol* (CBD) and many other chemicals. Prescription cannabinoid pills are approved by the U.S. Food and Drug Administration (FDA) for treating nausea and decreased appetite related to cancer or HIV. The only cannabinoid approved specifically for pain is a chemical constituent of marijuana called *nabiximols*, an extract containing both THC and CBD, which is marketed in Canada for pain due to multiple sclerosis. As for use in nerve pain, the data are conflicting. The side effects of oral and smoked marijuana, as well as varied legality in different states, complicate the issue.

The role of chelation therapy in people with elevated blood levels of metals, such as mercury and lead, is also controversial. In this treatment, a variety of chemicals, given orally or intravenously, bind to the metals, which are then excreted through the kidneys. If not done correctly, the treatment can cause kidney damage.

Treatment with Medication That Is Not a Pill

Some people get relief from topical medications, such as local anesthetics, applied as creams, sprays, or patches. Topical medications are best for small local areas of mild to moderately severe pain. Lidocaine is available as a cream, gel, or patch. Low doses of the cream or gel are available over the counter, but the Lidoderm patch, which contains 5 percent lidocaine, is by prescription. The patch is applied to the skin for no more than twelve hours a day. It is useful to relieve pain and tingling in small areas of skin, such as on the feet. EMLA (eutectic mixture of local anesthetics) cream is an over-the-counter topical medication that contains two local anesthetics, lidocaine and prilocaine. This cream may be useful for occasional application to small areas of skin.

Benzocaine spray is a local anesthetic that is available over the counter. It is marketed for relief of sunburn pain. All topical anesthetics have the same precautions. They are not recommended for use on large areas of skin or where there are breaks in the skin because the ingredients can be absorbed into the blood and cause side effects, the most worrisome being heart rhythm abnormalities and seizures. In those with liver dysfunction, even a small amount of anesthetic entering the bloodstream will not be properly metabolized and can build up in the blood.

Capsaicin, a chemical found in hot chili peppers, can provide pain relief. It is available over the counter as a low-concentration ointment, gel, or liquid, and by prescription as a higher concentration patch. It works by causing axon endings to release substance P, which mediates pain. The first application of capsaicin will cause pain as substance P flows out of axons, but repeated use will deplete substance P. A topical anesthetic cream, such as lidocaine or EMLA, with or without oral pain medications, is used before the first application of topical capsaicin. It is important to use capsaicin three to four times a day. If used less frequently, substance P will build up again in the axon endings, and each application will result in pain. Possible side effects of capsaicin use include elevated blood pressure as well as redness and pain at the site of application.

Recent evidence suggests that botulinum toxin type A may relieve neuropathic pain. The toxin blocks the release of acetylcholine from motor axons at the junction between the nerve and the muscle, causing muscle weakness. Botulinum toxin may also block the release of substances from sensory neurons that make nerves more sensitive to painful stimulation. In the studies that have been published, a very small dose is injected under the skin over the top of the feet in a grid pattern. Since the dose is quite low, the risk of causing muscle weakness in the feet is also low. Another possible side effect is bruising from the injection. Botulinum toxin injections typically have to be repeated every few months.

Medications

OK, we are doctors—we give pills. There are dozens of oral medications used for nerve pain. Some are FDA approved for use in nerve pain, and others are approved for other uses but have been shown, anecdotally, to help with pain. The American Academy of Neurology has produced evidence-based guidelines for the treatment of painful neuropathy. The guidelines, written for patients, can be found at www.aan.com/Guidelines/Home /GetGuidelineContent/481. Even though the guidelines refer to neuropathy caused by diabetes, they are useful for all types of painful neuropathy.

Medications can relieve the burning, prickling, and tingling of neuropathic pain. They belong to various classes of medicines, the two most common being antidepressants and antiseizure medications. Most of these medicines are not indicated by the FDA for treatment of nerve pain. Some have been noted to work anecdotally, and some have been studied but without going through the formal indication process required by the FDA. Currently, only two medications are indicated by the FDA for the treatment of nerve pain: pregabalin and duloxetine. They are specifically approved for use in nerve pain caused by diabetes, because the drugs were studied in people with diabetes-related neuropathy, but both are used for nerve pain caused by other conditions.

In the following sections, the number of milligrams listed is specific for each medication. Milligrams are not comparable between different medications. For example, 100 milligrams of one medicine is not the same as 100 milligrams of another.

Antidepressants

The use of an antidepressant for nerve pain does not mean that you are depressed. This is a different use for the medicine. Within this category, two subgroups are used for neuropathic pain: tricyclic antidepressants (named for their chemical structure) and selective serotonin and norepinephrine reuptake inhibitors (SSNRIs). Both classes of antidepressants increase the amount of active serotonin and norepinephrine in the brain. Serotonin and norepinephrine are neurotransmitters in the brain. Neurotransmitters are chemicals that transmit information from one neuron to another. Tricyclic antidepressants may also block the flow of current along the axon, decreasing the probability that an axon will fire.

Tricyclic antidepressants include amitriptyline, nortriptyline, and desipramine, among others. They are usually well tolerated and typically taken once or twice a day. These antidepressants may cause drowsiness, which could be desirable in those who have difficulty falling asleep. The side effects of tricyclic antidepressants are similar to the symptoms of autonomic nerve damage and can make those symptoms worse. These side effects include lightheadedness, dry eyes, dry mouth, sweating, difficulty urinating, constipation, and erectile dysfunction. In some people, these medicines can cause heart rhythm abnormalities. Drowsiness in elderly patients can lead to mental confusion and falls. Nortriptyline and desipramine may have fewer side effects than amitriptyline.

Typical doses of tricyclic antidepressants for use in nerve pain are listed below. (Note that the rate of dose increase for all medications described in this book will be determined for you, individually, by your physician.)

- Amitriptyline: a 10 to 25 mg tablet before bed as a starting dose, increasing to 75 to 100 mg as necessary. The maximum dose is 300 mg/day, but it is rarely used at such a high dose for nerve pain.
- Nortriptyline: a 10 to 25 mg capsule before bed as a starting dose, increasing to 75 to 100 mg as necessary. It may be split into two daily doses. The maximum dose is 150 mg/day. This is typically lower in the elderly.
- Desipramine: a 25 to 50 mg tablet before bed, increasing as necessary. The dose may be split into two daily doses. Maximum dose is 300 mg/day in nonelderly adults, and 150 mg/day in the elderly.

Duloxetine is an antidepressant medication of the SSNRI type. A typical starting dose is a 20 or 30 mg capsule before bed. If the medication is tolerated, it may be increased to a full standard dose of 60 mg within a week or two. Side effects may include drowsiness, dizziness, nausea, dry mouth, constipation, gastrointestinal upset, and increased sweating. There are rare reports of elevated blood pressure and liver dysfunction, so this medication should not be used in people with uncontrolled high blood pressure or liver disease. Another antidepressant in the same class, but without an FDA indication for nerve pain, is venlafaxine; some physicians prescribe this antidepressant for nerve pain as well. This medication has a long-acting form that may be better tolerated than duloxetine. It can have the same type of side effects as duloxetine. A common dose is 37.5 mg in tablet or capsule form once or twice a day, with a maximum of 225 mg a day in divided doses.

Almost all antidepressant drugs come with a warning of increased feelings of suicidality in some people, although this is an uncommon effect. Your doctor will talk with you about this if she prescribes antidepressants for your nerve pain.

Antiseizure Medication

Prescribing an antiseizure medicine for your nerve pain does not mean that the doctor thinks you have seizures or epilepsy. Pregabalin capsules have a separate approval by the FDA for the treatment of nerve pain. A typical starting dose is 75 mg once a day, with a maximum daily dose of 300 mg in divided doses.

Gabapentin is a related medication that is commonly used for nerve pain because it is effective, well tolerated, and inexpensive, even though this use is not indicated by the FDA. A typical starting dose is a 100 to 300 mg capsule or tablet before bed, slowly increasing in dose and in frequency to two or three times a day. Gabapentin often requires a dose of between 900 and 3,600 mg a day to provide relief. A long-acting form is available.

Both pregabalin and gabapentin act on the brain and the nerves to reduce pain. For both medications, the most common side effect is drowsiness, which can be mitigated by starting at a low dose and increasing slowly. Other possible side effects include dizziness, weight gain, headache, dry mouth, and swelling in the legs. Very high doses may cause muscle twitching.

Older antiseizure medications such as phenytoin and carbamazepine are used much less frequently because of their side effects. Sedatives and muscle relaxers, such as carisoprodol (Soma), are not recommended because of their lack of efficacy for nerve pain and their potential for addiction.

When discussing which pain medication is best for you, your doctor will take into consideration your other medical problems, allergies, and medications you are taking. Disease of the liver or kidneys may require a change in dosage. Medicines can be used alone or in combination. Make sure to ask your doctor how long it should take before you notice an effect of the medication. Should it help with the first dose or do you have to build up a certain level of medication in your system? Your doctor will discuss the medication schedule.

Timing of pain medications is essential. The goal is to take each dose before the pain starts again. It is important to ask these questions: Should I take it as soon as I wake up to give the medication time to work before starting the day? Should I take pain medication at night to help me sleep? Are there foods to avoid? What if I miss a dose? Ask about side effects and the most efficient way to reach your doctor with questions. Does the use of this medication require monitoring, and if so, what type and how often? For example, in some instances you need blood or urine tests or an electrocardiogram before starting the medication. Sometimes it all boils down to deciding which dosing regimen and side effects sound best to you.

What If Nothing Works?

Most people get good relief with the techniques and medications described in this chapter. If oral medications are not effective, the first step is to look again at what is causing the pain. Perhaps the cause is not neuropathy but some other problem that needs to be treated differently. If no other cause is found, then referral to a physician who specializes in pain control is appropriate. These specialized physicians are expert at less common treatments for nerve pain. These treatments may include narcotic medication given orally or through a patch worn on the skin; intravenous (into the vein) infusions of anesthetic-like medication; or rarely, implantation of a device that gives electrical stimulation to the spinal cord to block pain signals coming from the nerves before they reach the brain.

The use of opioid medication (narcotics) for neuropathic pain is controversial. It is not a first-line treatment. These medications include morphine, tramadol, oxycodone, and hydrocodone, either alone or in combination with an anti-inflammatory medicine such as aspirin, acetaminophen, or naproxen. Experts generally agree that chronic pain should be treated with long-acting narcotics rather than short-acting formulations. With short-acting medication, the medicine wears off, you develop pain, and then need another dose, a cycle that is uncomfortable and cumbersome. It is better to keep the pain at bay than to live a life of cyclic pain and relief. Rarely, a small dose of a short-acting opioid before bed is useful for those whose pain makes it difficult to fall asleep and who have not had relief with other types of medication.

No evidence shows that opioid pain medication provides significant pain relief for more than a few months at a time. As with all narcotics, there is the risk of dependence. Side effects include drowsiness, constipation, withdrawal, and depressed breathing, as well as the complications that can arise from other people abusing your medication. Tolerance for the euphoric and pain-relieving effects of opioids precedes tolerance for respiratory depression, which can decrease the drive to breathe. This is particularly dangerous when opioid medication is combined with others that depress respiration, including benzodiazepines (such as Valium, Xanax, and Ativan) and sedatives such as barbiturates and alcohol. The American Academy of Neurology has published a position paper regarding the use of narcotic medication for pain, "Opioids for Chronic Noncancer Pain," which can be found by searching for the title on the AAN website, www.aan.com.

Treatment of Motor Neuropathy Symptoms

Cramps, weakness, and muscle wasting are the most common problems with motor neuropathy. For cramps, stretching the muscles for fifteen minutes before bed is often recommended, although there is no evidence that it helps. Dehydration may increase the frequency of cramps, so staying well hydrated is important. There is some evidence that B complex vitamin supplements and a blood pressure medication called diltiazem may help some people with muscle cramps. Oral magnesium supplementation can be useful, especially for people taking proton-pump inhibitors to treat stomach ulcers and esophageal reflux.

Common medications in this category are omeprazole (Prilosec), esomeprazole (Nexium), lansoprazole (Prevacid), and others. Talk to your doctor about the correct dose of magnesium for you. In the past, quinine was used to prevent muscle cramps, but it caused serious side effects in a small number of people, including blood clots and low blood-platelet counts. It is now approved by the FDA solely for treatment of malaria. Even the amount of quinine in tonic water can have adverse effects, so drinking tonic water is not recommended for preventing muscle cramps.

Physical and Occupational Therapy

Your doctor may prescribe physical therapy, gait training, and occupational therapy. Physical therapy deals with improving or maintaining strength, balance, and endurance. Gait training helps specifically with balance and walking. Occupational therapy focuses on improving the use of the hands and arms.

Muscles depend on their nerve supply to stay healthy and strong. With neuropathy, building muscle mass and strength is difficult. With the help of physical therapy, however, it is possible to maintain the strength that you have. Recent clinical trials have demonstrated that regular exercise may lead to improvement of symptoms in people with diabetic neuropathy. This improvement may be due to more than the effect of exercise on blood sugar control alone. In addition, tai chi can help improve balance, and yoga can improve flexibility. Autonomic neuropathy can interfere with heart function and blood pressure maintenance, so speak with your doctor before starting a course of exercise. A physical therapist can design a program that is right for you. Physical therapy, gait training, and balance exercises combined may be the most effective non-medication-based intervention for people with neuropathy. If walking is difficult because of an inability to lift the feet, physical therapy can also assist with devices to help hold the foot steady and with leg braces, if needed.

Occupational therapy includes exercises to help maintain the strength of the hands, but the therapist can also recommend devices to assist with daily activities, such as writing, typing, and using utensils. Physical and occupational therapists can both evaluate your home and give recommendations for modifications and devices to make life easier. These include things like stairway lifts; bathroom grab bars; raised toilet seats; easy-entry showers; modified kitchen utensils, pens, and toothbrushes; and clothes with easy-to-manipulate closures.

Treatment of Autonomic Symptoms

Often the underlying cause of autonomic neuropathy is not responsive to treatment. Even if sensory and motor symptoms improve, sometimes autonomic symptoms do not. Autonomic axons are very thin and do not have a firm connective tissue tube to grow through, so it is difficult for them to grow back after being damaged. Treatment of symptoms is often the best your doctor can offer.

Treatment of Lightheadedness

Feeling faint or lightheaded (*orthostatic hypotension*) can be one of the most difficult and dangerous symptoms of autonomic neuropathy. A fall can cause injury and be particularly dangerous if it occurs on stairs or while crossing the street. Before such symptoms are ascribed to neuropathy, however, other causes must be investigated, such as abnormal heart rhythm or dehydration. Lightheadedness is treated with a combination of lifestyle changes and medications. Lifestyle changes include rising slowly from beds and chairs; contracting the large muscles in the legs before standing up, to decrease the pooling of blood in the legs; and not straining during bowel movements or urination, both of which can lower blood pressure. Elevating the head of your bed while sleeping will raise your blood pressure a bit in the mornings, which may help with lightheadedness. Dietary changes include good hydration and increased salt intake, if this is permitted by your doctor. Salt is necessary to keep the fluid you drink inside blood vessels, so drinking water alone will not do the trick. Large meals divert blood to the gastrointestinal tract and away from other organs. Smaller, more frequent meals may be better tolerated. Alcohol will cause dehydration and dilation of blood vessels, both lowering blood pressure. Discussion of this symptom with your doctor along with routine blood pressure measurements may lead to a decrease in dose or a discontinuation of medication for high blood pressure. Compression stockings are sometimes suggested, but they need to be thigh-high stockings to be useful, which can be cumbersome and uncomfortable. Compression stockings that go to the knee can compress a nerve that runs around the knee and innervates the muscles that lift up the foot and toes. These stockings can cause nerve damage in addition to the underlying cause and are to be avoided.

Medications commonly used to treat lightheadedness consist of those that increase the volume of the blood and those that cause blood vessels to constrict, which raises blood pressure. Fludrocortisone is in the first category. It causes the kidneys to reabsorb water, increasing the amount of water in blood vessels, which raises blood pressure. A common starting dose is 0.1 mg a day, with a maximum of 0.3 mg a day. This drug would not be used in someone with heart failure because it presents the heart with more blood to pump, making the organ work harder. Midodrine and a newer agent, droxidopa, are in the second category. The standard dose for midodrine is 2.5 to 10 mg taken up to three times a day, with a maximum dose of 0.3 mg a day, and for droxidopa, a 100 mg capsule three times a day, with a maximum of 1,800 mg a day. All these medications can cause blood pressure to be too high when you are lying down. Your doctor will have to adjust the dose to strike the right balance between blood pressure that is too low and too high.

Sweating

Autonomic nerves innervate the sweat glands, causing you to sweat when it is hot in order to maintain a normal body temperature. With neuropathy, sweating decreases in the areas of skin that are numb and painful and increases in other areas. It may feel like you are sweating more than usual on your head, underarms, and trunk. Managing this symptom includes wearing clothes in layers you can remove as necessary to keep cool and avoiding hot environments where your body temperature may rise. If focal areas of sweating are difficult to handle, small areas can be treated with topical antiperspirants or botulinum toxin injections, which will stop the nerves from signaling the glands to produce sweat.

Adjustment of the Eyes to Light

Autonomic nerves regulate how much light enters the eye by causing the pupils to open wide in dim light and to constrict in bright light. If transitioning from darkness to a bright environment is uncomfortable, you can make the transition slowly, giving time for your eyes to adjust, or use sunglasses that block ultraviolet light.

Bladder Symptoms

As discussed in chapter 3, neuropathy may lead to a flaccid bladder that does not contract with normal force. With autonomic neuropathy, you may no longer feel when your bladder is full, so that you do not know when you need to urinate. When you do urinate, autonomic neuropathy can cause decreased contraction of the bladder, with incomplete emptying. Incomplete bladder emptying and loss of sensation lead to an overfilled and enlarged bladder, which may leak spontaneously or with coughing, laughing, or running. An overfilled bladder may lead to urinary tract and kidney infections. Scheduled trips to the bathroom can help avoid overfilling the bladder and the subsequent leakage of urine. Setting the alarm on your clock or phone for two- to four-hour intervals will remind you to urinate, even if you don't feel as though you need to.

You can also practice techniques that help with urination, such as the Credé maneuver and Valsalva voiding, which use your abdominal muscles to assist with urination. The Credé maneuver involves applying pressure over the lower abdomen with the hands during urination. This maneuver has two steps. While standing in front of or sitting on the toilet, place your hands palms down, flat on your abdomen, below the belly button. Push firmly in and downward five or six times. This should result in some urination. Then place one hand on top of the other and move down to the pubic area. Again, press firmly inward and downward to expel the last bit of urine. If you can, contract the abdominal muscles to apply more pressure during both maneuvers. The Valsalva maneuver consists of breathing out with force against a closed airway, for example, while holding the nostrils closed or preventing air from leaving the throat. Valsalva voiding involves leaning forward to increase pressure on the abdomen, or bearing down as though you are having a bowel movement while breathing out forcefully against a closed throat. This increases pressure on the bladder and leads to more complete emptying.

If voiding maneuvers are not successful, *catheterization* will be necessary to empty the bladder. In catheterization, a thin, flexible latex or silicone catheter (tube) is placed into the bladder through the urethra in order to drain the bladder. The urethra is the tube that runs from the bladder to the outside. In men the urethra runs through the penis; in women it exits just above the vaginal opening.

Catheterization can be intermittent or indwelling. For intermittent catheterization, a one-use-only catheter is placed, under clean conditions, through the urethra and into the bladder. The urine is drained and the catheter removed. You and a caregiver would be trained to do this. It can be uncomfortable, especially when you are new at it. A slippery gel on the catheter makes it easier to insert and decreases discomfort. You and your doctor will come up with the best schedule for you. Just as with scheduled voiding, setting an alarm will remind you to catheterize and avoid an overfilled bladder and the problems that go along with it.

The main type of indwelling bladder catheter is the Foley catheter. This is a thin, flexible tube with a balloon on the end that gets inserted into the bladder. The catheter is inserted through the urethra, into the bladder, and then the balloon is inflated with saline, using a needleless syringe through a side port on the tube. The inflated balloon in the bladder keeps the catheter from falling out. The free end of the catheter can be attached to a collection bag, which can be worn on the leg, or the catheter can be clamped and drained intermittently. To remove the catheter, simply deflate the balloon and slip the catheter out. Advantages of an indwelling catheter like the Foley include a stable catheter that can stay in place for as long as one month before being changed, without the repeated trauma to the urethra caused by intermittent catheters. The schedule will be different for each person, depending on the risk of infection and the risk of clogging of the catheter. In addition to possible infection or irritation of the urethra, disadvantages include the inconvenience of wearing a collection bag as well as the risk of the catheter falling out. There are different types of indwelling catheters, and your doctor will discuss which is best for you. You and your caregiver will be taught how to use the catheter.

If performing catheterization is not possible because of dexterity or cognitive problems, surgical placement of a catheter is an option. Using local or general anesthesia, the surgeon inserts the catheter above the belly button, directly through the abdominal wall and into the bladder, then secures it in place so it will not fall out. This is called a *suprapubic catheter*. The external end of the catheter is attached to a collection bag or can be clamped and used for scheduled voiding. Advantages of this method include avoiding damage to the urethra (and penis in men), easier hygiene, and easier access for sexual activity. The procedure is reversible—the exit site will heal when the tube is removed. Disadvantages include the need for a doctor to change the tube every month or so, risk of infection, and, for those with obesity, difficulty draining the tube while sitting. Rarely, more invasive surgical techniques are used to create catheter access to the bladder through the abdominal wall. Your neurologist will refer you to a urologist to discuss the best treatment option for you.

Unfortunately, no medications stimulate the bladder to contract. Bethanechol has been useful in experimental conditions, but it is not used clinically. One class of medication, called α-blockers (meaning they block the α-adrenergic receptor found on various tissues), can relax the bladder sphincter muscle and ease the outflow of urine. Examples of these medications include tamsulosin hydrochloride and terazosin. Side effects of these medications can include dizziness, headache, and fatigue. SSNRIs, the class of antidepressant medications discussed above, are also used to relax the bladder sphincter. Every medication has side effects, and proper use of these medications for bladder dysfunction is best discussed with a urologist.

Gastrointestinal Symptoms

Autonomic neuropathy can cause slowing down or speeding up of the gastrointestinal tract. It may take more time for food to move through the stomach and less time for it to move through the intestine. Swallowing may be difficult because of slowed movement of food down the esophagus. Acid reflux from the stomach into the lower esophagus may occur as a result of weakness of the sphincter muscle between the esophagus and the stomach. Changes in eating patterns can help with gastrointestinal symptoms. Meals that are high in fat stay in the stomach longer. When food stays in the stomach for too long, it is absorbed erratically, which can cause swings in blood sugar levels. Eating more frequent, smaller meals that are low in fat may prevent nausea and bloating as well as possibly decreasing the severity of diarrhea. A high-fiber diet can also help with diarrhea. Some foods, such as chocolate and alcohol, may increase acid reflux. Going to sleep on an empty stomach and sleeping with the head of the bed elevated a small bit can decrease acid reflux.

Metoclopramide, 5 to 20 mg taken thirty minutes before meals and before bed, can speed up stomach emptying and calm nausea, but it can also make diarrhea worse. Paradoxically, agents that increase movement of the intestine can help people struggling with alternating diarrhea and constipation.

Diarrhea can be treated with medications that slow the movement of the intestines. These include over-the-counter opioid derivatives, such as loperamide and diphenoxylate with atropine. Loperamide is taken in divided doses of 4 to 8 mg a day. Diphenoxylate/atropine is given as a dose of 5/0.05 to 20/0.05 mg a day. Side effects of both include drowsiness and dry mouth. Tincture of opium is another agent in this family. It requires a prescription and comes as a liquid, with the dose measured in milliliters. Your physician would decide the dose that is best for you.

Sexual Dysfunction

Neuropathy can directly and indirectly cause various problems with sexual intercourse for both men and women. Indirectly, pain, medication side effects, and lifestyle changes related to neuropathy can interfere with libido. Nerve damage itself, as well as medication effects, can interfere with erection and ejaculation in men and vaginal lubrication and orgasm in women.

The Special Treatment Needs of Men

Erectile dysfunction is common with autonomic neuropathy and is often one of the first symptoms. Treatment may involve medication or other techniques. Autonomic nerves in the penis release an unusual neurotransmitter, nitrous oxide, the same "laughing gas" you get at the dentist. Nitrous oxide causes dilation of veins, which leads to erection. If there are not enough axons to release enough nitrous oxide, this won't occur. Medications such as sildenafil, tadalafil, and vardenafil work by inhibiting the breakdown of nitrous oxide after it is released by axons. Nitrous oxide then stays around and functions for a bit longer. These medications will not work unless some autonomic nerve function remains.

Alprostadil, a prostaglandin that causes dilation of blood vessels, is given by injection into the penis or by urethral suppository. This medication may be used alone or in various combinations with papaverine and phentolamine. Nondrug interventions include structural implants and vacuum devices to draw blood into the penis.

Erectile dysfunction may have other causes as well, including disease of blood vessels, which is common in high blood pressure and diabetes; sensory neuropathy with decreased penile sensation; and psychological factors, such as depression and anxiety. Sexual dysfunction is a constantly evolving field, so it is important to get an opinion from a urologist who specializes in erectile dysfunction.

The Special Treatment Needs of Women

Nerves innervating the vagina cause glands to release lubricating fluids before intercourse. If these nerves are damaged, vaginal dryness and subsequent pain with intercourse will result. In postmenopausal women, estrogen cream can relieve dryness. Over-the-counter lubricants, such as Astroglide and Slippery Stuff, will also ease dryness. As in men, nerves that release nitrous oxide lead to increased blood flow, which in women causes engorgement of the clitoris. Thus, nerve damage can interfere with orgasm. Currently, there is no consensus about the use of sildenafil-like medications for sexual dysfunction in women.

For both genders, communicating openly and honestly as well as taking it slow can help to overcome some of these problems. Consultation with a gynecologist and a urologist who specialize in sexual issues can be useful.

Future Treatments

Medications that protect nerves from damage caused by other medications as well as medicines that reverse nerve damage caused by illnesses are currently under development. In the future, you may receive a medication to protect your nerves against the effects of drugs that can cause neuropathy. This may be particularly true for chemotherapy drugs used to treat cancer. In addition, your doctor may also be able to prescribe medication to reverse neuropathy caused by illness.

Alternative Treatments

Unfortunately, some people seek financial gain by selling unproven and useless cures and treatments for illnesses. This practice is particularly rampant on the Internet. You'll find various supplements, electrical devices, and even surgery to decompress nerves, all touted to treat neuropathy, despite no proven positive effect on the underlying causes or symptoms of the condition. One device advertised on the Internet consists of a plastic bucket and a battery, with sticky pads on the ends of its wires. You put water in the plastic bucket, stick the pads on your feet, put your feet in the water, then give your feet electrical shocks from the battery—all for a mere seven hundred dollars! Anodyne light therapy is also touted as a treatment for nerve pain. This treatment shines light on the feet, dilating blood vessels and, indeed, possibly making you feel better as it warms your feet. But this same outcome can be had by sitting in the sun or putting your feet in warm water, which is much less expensive than a six-thousand-dollar machine or a series of expensive clinic treatments! Attention should be paid to the wording of any advertisement for a device. To acquire *clearance* from the FDA to market a medical device, the applicant must show only that the device is "substantially equivalent" to a device that is already legally marketed for the same use. To be *approved* by the FDA, however, the applicant must provide reasonable assurance of the device's safety and effectiveness.

Some supplements, such as alpha-lipoic acid, linolenic acid (contained in primrose oil), and Neuracel, are advertised as helpful for nerve pain. These claims are all unproven, and the supplements are usually quite expensive. Multiple clinical trials with alpha-lipoic acid have been inconclusive. Currently, the FDA is forbidden by law to regulate supplements unless they have been shown to cause harm. Recent investigations in New York state have found a high proportion of supplements on the market that contain none of the advertised ingredient or that contain the ingredient at a dose different from what is listed on the bottle. In addition, supplements may contain fillers that are not listed on the label and to which some people may be allergic. Some supplements can interact negatively with prescription medications. Others may contain dangerously high amounts of vitamin B6. Ayurvedic medicines are not regulated and have been found in the past to be contaminated with lead, mercury, and arsenic. Supplements, homeopathic medications, and Ayurvedic treatments advertised for nerve health or nerve pain are not recommended. You can find more information about the effects and safety of specific supplements in the About Herbs database at www.mskcc.org/aboutherbs.

CHAPTER 8

Clinical Trials

When I was asked to be in a clinical trial, I first thought about how it would help me. Then I thought about how it could help other people. I have come to understand that though the odds of the new treatment helping me were small, it could likely help other people, which is all right with me. I was afraid that I would get the placebo, but this was the only trial available to me, so I was glad to take the chance. I also accepted the risk of side effects. Which was worse, possible side effects or the missed opportunity to get a medicine that could help? Plus, I knew that when the study was over, I would receive the real medication. Traveling to the hospital frequently was a hardship, but I knew it was what I had to do. After the study was published, I was told I had been in the placebo group, but when I read the results—the medication worked—I was glad I had participated.

Clinical trials are scientific experiments with new medications or procedures. For patients with neuropathy, there are clinical trials for treatments of the causes of neuropathy as well as for treatments of nerve pain. Your doctor may ask if you are interested in participating in a clinical trial.

These trials occur in three phases. During phase 1, the new medication is given to a small number of healthy volunteers. This happens after the medication has been tested on animals. The purpose of a phase 1 trial is to determine the medication's safety, which includes looking for side effects, and to determine an appropriate dose. In addition, phase 1 trials enable researchers to study how human subjects metabolize the new drug.

Phase 2 trials typically involve small groups of patients with the condition or symptoms that the medication is intended to treat. These trials are conducted in one of two ways. Either all the patients are given the active drug or some patients are given the active drug, and others are not. In the second case, the groups are determined randomly. The purpose of this phase is to continue evaluating the safety of the drug as well as to get an idea of the drug's effectiveness. These trials have too few participants to provide results that are conclusive enough to allow for approval by the U.S. Food and Drug Administration (FDA).

Phase 3 trials are called *double-blind, randomized placebo-controlled trials*. These are the gold standard of clinical trials, the studies that the FDA uses to decide whether to approve a new medication for sale in the United States. *Double blind* means that neither the study participants nor the investigators know who is getting medicine and who is getting placebo. A placebo (from the Latin word meaning "I shall please") is a substance with no medicinal activity—a sugar pill. *Randomized placebo controlled* means that patients are randomly chosen to get active medication or placebo. This is done by a computer program that assigns patients as they enter the study. In some studies, half the patients get the drug and half get the placebo; in others, the ratio is different, with more patients receiving the active drug than the placebo. The active medication and placebo look alike and are given in the same way so that the patients and investigators do not know who is getting which treatment. In some trials, the new medication is compared to an older medication rather than to placebo. Each trial will have different rules about what medications you can take while on the trial. This will be explained in detail during the informed consent process.

For some patients, the idea of receiving an unproved drug is difficult to accept and requires trust in the scientific method. People worry that they are "guinea pigs." You will never be placed in a clinical trial without your formal informed consent. Universities and other institutions that perform clinical trials are overseen by a Human Subjects Institutional Review Board that must give permission for any clinical trial to begin. You will be given an informed consent form, which will be reviewed with you in detail. You will be told the purpose of the study, the name of the medication, any blood work or testing that is required, all possible known side effects, the ratio of patients who will receive active medication to those who will received placebo, and the method by which the medication or placebo will be administered. The form will require your signature before any part of the trial can be started. If you decline to participate, there will be no negative consequences. It can be scary to know that you might not receive the active drug. Remember that you may withdraw from any trial at any time for any reason. Travel to the trial site can be expensive and time consuming. These issues will be discussed with you during the informed consent process. Travel, hotel, and meal expenses may be paid by the drug company.

All clinical trials have an independent Data Safety and Review Board, made up of investigators from outside the testing institution. The members of this board are the only people who know which patients are receiving the active drug and which are receiving placebo. To look out for the safety of study participants, the board reviews study data periodically to make sure that the group receiving the active drug is not experiencing more frequent or serious side effects than those receiving placebo. The board also looks to see if patients getting the active drug are doing so much better than those receiving placebo that it is no longer ethical to continue the study. In this case, the study is stopped early, and all patients in the trial may receive the active drug.

At the end of the phase 3 trial, the data are analyzed and a report is submitted to the FDA. The study is also typically published in a medical journal. The process from phase 1 to phase 3 and FDA approval of a drug takes many years. The wait can be frustrating and even infuriating to patients who may benefit from a new medication, but this process is necessary to demonstrate the effectiveness and safety of new medications. Because of this long time course, patients in clinical trials may not benefit directly from the trial. This will also be explained to you prior to your signing an informed consent form. The good news is that in many trials, each study participant is given the active drug when he or she completes the trial.

CHAPTER 9

Other Conditions That Feel Like Neuropathy

There is no differential diagnosis in Neurology. There is what it is and what it isn't.

Attributed to Raymond Adams, MD (1911–2008)

All that tingles is not peripheral neuropathy. Part of your doctor's evaluation of your condition includes considering illnesses that look or feel like peripheral neuropathy but are not. In this chapter, I describe illnesses that can be mistaken for neuropathy.

Radiculopathy and Radiculitis

Damage to the sensory and motor nerve roots can cause pain and weakness. This is a condition called *radiculopathy*. The nerve roots can be damaged a number of ways. The motor and sensory roots can be compressed by bony overgrowth caused by arthritis in the back or by a herniated intervertebral disc (when a disc in the spine bulges out). Pinched nerves exiting the lower back can cause pain and numbness in the feet and weakness in the legs.

Damage to motor and sensory roots can also be caused by inflammation. This is called *radiculitis*. The symptoms are the same as with radiculopathy. Lyme disease, caused by the bacterium *Borrelia burgdorferi*, does not cause typical axonal neuropathy but does cause radiculitis. *Herpes zoster*, the virus that causes chickenpox, also causes inflammation of sensory nerves along a small area of skin. When this occurs, it is called *shingles*. Both of these processes can be mistaken for peripheral neuropathy.

Your doctor should be able to tell the difference between radiculopathy, radiculitis, and peripheral neuropathy based on your history of symptoms as well as the neurological examination and tests, such as blood work, MRI of the lower back, nerve conduction studies, and electromyography.

Carpal Tunnel Syndrome

Carpal tunnel syndrome is a common condition that can be mistaken for a generalized neuropathy. It is caused by compression of the *median nerve,* a nerve that runs down the arm, under a band of connective tissue that wraps around the wrist and extends into the thumb and next three fingers. Carpal tunnel syndrome has many possible underlying causes, the most common being diabetes mellitus, pregnancy, and thyroid disease, but it can also develop without an obvious cause. Carpal tunnel syndrome may be associated with repetitive motion of the wrist and hands. The syndrome comprises symptoms in the thumb, index finger, middle finger, and sometimes half of the ring finger. These symptoms include tingling, pain, numbness, as well as feeling as though the hand is swollen. Sometimes there is weakness of the muscles that move the thumb, resulting in difficulty with opening jars, fastening buttons, and picking up small objects with the thumb and index finger.

People often notice symptoms at night that wake them from sleep, as well as when driving a car or performing other motions that involve bending the wrist. Symptoms become noticeable with these activities because they cause compression of the nerve. Although carpal tunnel syndrome is not the same as peripheral neuropathy, the two sometimes occur together. Diagnosis is determined by history, examination, and sometimes the use of nerve conduction studies and electromyography. Treatment of carpal tunnel syndrome ranges from using a wrist splint at night or taking aspirinlike medication to receiving steroid injections in the wrist or having surgery.

Muscle Disease

Diseases of muscle can produce slowly progressive weakness in the legs, which can be mistaken for peripheral neuropathy. Unlike neuropathy, however, muscle disease does not produce numbness, tingling, or a pins-and-needles sort of pain. A good medical history, examination, blood tests, and NCS/EMG can reliably differentiate between disease of muscle and disease of nerves.

Diseases of the Central Nervous System

The nervous system is divided into the central nervous system and the peripheral nervous system. The central nervous system comprises the brain and spinal cord. Nerve roots coming out of the spinal cord, nerves in the limbs and trunk, and muscles make up the peripheral nervous system.

Diseases of the brain and spinal cord can have symptoms similar to peripheral neuropathy. One common neuropathy lookalike is multiple sclerosis, a demyelinating autoimmune disease of the central nervous system. The exact cause of multiple sclerosis is not known, but it is characterized by immune cells attacking the myelin in the brain and spinal cord. The myelin that surrounds axons in the peripheral nervous system is a bit different from the myelin that surrounds axons in the central nervous system. The two forms of myelin are not made by the same cells, and they differ chemically from each other. In the central nervous system, myelin is made by cells called *oligodendrocytes*; in the peripheral nervous system, Schwann cells produce myelin. Talking about demyelinating neuropathy and demyelinating disease of the central nervous system, like multiple sclerosis, as two distinct diseases can be confusing, but they are different diseases. The myelin is not the same in these diseases, and neither are the antibodies that cause damage. Having one does not increase your risk of having the other.

Multiple sclerosis can start with numbness or weakness in one part of the body. The onset of symptoms usually occurs quickly, in a matter of hours to days, as opposed to neuropathy, which progresses over weeks to years. In addition, the symptoms of multiple sclerosis appear over large patches of the body; for example, the sudden onset of numbness or weakness in one arm, one leg, or the trunk on one side of the body. Peripheral axonal neuropathy comes on more slowly, and the symptoms are symmetrical and length dependent, starting in the feet. A careful history, examination, MRI of the brain and spinal cord as well as examination of cerebrospinal fluid can reliably differentiate multiple sclerosis and other diseases of the central nervous system from peripheral neuropathy.

Metabolic Diseases

Rarely, diseases of the liver, gallbladder, or kidney can cause itching and tingling in the arms and legs as a result of waste product buildup in the blood. When the liver is not working as it should, or when the gallbladder is diseased, *bilirubin*—a breakdown product of red blood cells—builds up in the blood. When the kidneys are not working as they should, *urea*—a breakdown product of protein—builds up in the blood. Both substances can cause skin irritation and symptoms similar to peripheral neuropathy. Both can be tested for in the blood.

Though diabetes mellitus can cause a slowly progressing neuropathy, rapid lowering of very high blood sugar can cause transient symptoms of neuropathy that typically stop when blood sugar is sustained at a normal level.

Syphilis

Syphilis is caused by infection with the bacterium *Treponema pallidum*. Untreated syphilis can spread to the spinal cord and to the sensory neurons along the spinal cord. Damage to these structures causes electrical shooting pain in the legs, called *lightning pains*, and difficulty walking because joint position sensation is lacking. These symptoms can be mistaken for neuropathy. This pain and loss of coordination from untreated syphilis, called *tabes dorsalis*, is very rare today. It is treated with intravenous antibiotics.

CHAPTER 10

Living with Neuropathy

After my diagnosis of neuropathy, my doctor explained that I would have to do frequent inspections of my feet because I would not know if they had been cut or bruised. I was also told to file my toenails instead of cutting them. Well, I kept cutting them until one day, I cut a piece of skin off my big toe, which started to bleed. It did not hurt but just bled. I'm slow to learn some lessons, but now I file my nails when I complete my foot inspections. During another foot inspection, I noticed that one toenail was black. When my doctor looked at it, he asked how I had done it, and I did not know. I didn't remember how it happened. The black color was caused by blood built up under the nail. Good thing about neuropathy—I don't feel the throbbing pain when something like that happens. Sure enough, I did lose that nail, and I continue to inspect my feet daily.

The effects of neuropathy, including pain, numbness, weakness, autonomic dysfunction, and trouble with balance, can make basic activities of daily living difficult or impossible. Over time, people with neuropathy may have to depend on others for help with day-to-day activities, including transportation, cooking, cleaning, dressing, and personal hygiene. Understandably, this can lead to feelings of helplessness, frustration, depression, and anger. Your doctor is a source of information and referral to help you accommodate neuropathy-related changes in your function, mood, and personal relationships. Occupational and physical therapists can provide adaptive tools and techniques to maintain independence for as long as possible. Referral to a psychological or religious counselor is not a sign of weakness or shame; it is the mark of a strong person who does what needs to be done to achieve the best possible quality of life.

Neuropathy can be a lonely illness. You might look just fine, but the tingling, numbness, and burning are with you always. The effects of neuropathy might be difficult to discuss with others, who don't feel what you feel and who may not understand the reality of your symptoms. Support groups and online discussion groups may be helpful in contacting others with the same symptoms.

Sometimes there is shame in asking for help or medication. You may be afraid that the doctor will think you are a drug abuser, for example. Given the variety of medications now available specifically for nerve pain, your doctor may be able to control your pain without the use of narcotic medication. It is not necessary for you to suffer with nerve pain, and discussion with your doctor is the place to start to find some relief.

Caregivers sharing responsibilities and taking planned time away can help relieve stress for both the caregiver and the patient. Psychological therapy, without or with medication for depression or anxiety, can bring about understanding and a lighter mood. Many patients talk about their "new normal"—how they are at that moment. Mourning for what has been lost is normal. Understanding what can be accomplished and enjoyed at the "current normal" can bring peace of mind.

Lifestyle Changes

The two most important lifestyle changes to help keep nerves healthy are cutting back on alcohol and quitting smoking. Alcohol is toxic to neurons. Though an occasional glass of wine can add enjoyment to life, daily or heavy alcohol use can contribute to nerve damage. As for smoking, with every puff, the nicotine that enters the bloodstream leads to constriction of blood vessels throughout the body. This includes the blood vessels that nourish the nerves and the cells that support them. Alcohol and tobacco use can make neuropathy from other causes worse.

Other lifestyle changes that can help keep nerves healthy include daily exercise and eating a nutritious, well-rounded diet that includes fruits and vegetables. In addition, a good night's sleep may decrease the pain from neuropathy during the day.

Driving

Decreased sensation in the feet, weakness, and episodes of lightheadedness can impair your ability to drive. You need to be honest with yourself about your ability to drive safely, both for your own sake and for the sake of those around you. Modifications such as hand controls can keep you driving after foot controls become difficult to use. A physical therapist and your local Department of Motor Vehicles can give guidance regarding driving safety and automobile modifications.

Falls

Neuropathy pain, sensory loss, and weakness of the feet and legs increase the risk of falling. Falls are more likely when walking on an uneven or irregular surface. In older people, falling can lead to hip fracture. Physical therapy and walking aids can help reduce the risk of falls. Gait training is a specialized physical therapy technique that may improve balance and endurance.

Use of the Hands

As neuropathy progresses, it may be difficult to use your hands because of numbness, pain, and weakness. Occupational therapists are specially trained to aid in the use of hands and arms. Assistive devices, such as splints, utensils with wide handles, and devices to make computer and telephone use easier, can provide independence in some activities of daily living.

Foot Care

Foot care is sometimes the most important advice I give in the office. Neuropathy greatly increases the risk of toe and foot ulcers. The increased risk is due to a combination of factors, including lack of sensation to protect the feet, abnormalities of blood circulation, abnormal sweating, thinned skin, and poor wound healing. These complications usually occur later in the course of neuropathy and with severe neuropathies. When you lose the ability to feel pain and temperature in your feet, injury can occur without your being aware of it. Inability to feel temperature can lead to burns or frostbite. Small cuts and blisters will not be felt and can become infected. Antibiotics used for treatment of infection are carried in the blood to the infected toes, but neuropathy can decrease blood flow, making it difficult for the blood to deliver that antibiotic to the toes. Atrophy of foot muscles leads to weakness and difficulty maintaining the structure of the foot. This, coupled with a lack of joint sensation, can deform the foot. These changes, along with the poor blood flow and thin, dry skin caused by neuropathy, can lead to ulcers on the foot. If you can't feel your feet, you don't know if you are cutting skin when cutting your nails and you can't tell when the bath water is too hot.

Foot care consists of feeling bath water temperature with your hand; inspecting your feet and toes every day, looking for cuts or blisters; having someone else trim your toenails, filing rather than cutting nails; keeping the feet well moisturized to prevent cracking; not wearing shoes without socks or going barefoot; and wearing shoes that fit properly. A podiatrist or pedicurist who specializes in neuropathy can help keep feet healthy by trimming nails safely, inspecting shoe fit, and suggesting shoe inserts that add padding and redistribute pressure evenly throughout the foot to help prevent ulcers.

Ignoring toe and foot problems caused by neuropathy can lead to the need for amputation. If toes or feet become infected repeatedly, or antibiotic treatment is not effective, amputation is the only way to stop infection from spreading. This is why I emphasize the importance of foot care with all my patients. As I say many times a day, "I want you to have all ten toes, all the time."

A Word about Sex

Many patients are reluctant to discuss sex with their doctor. Don't be shy! Your doctor knows that neuropathy can interfere with sexual function but might be reluctant to ask you about it, especially if a spouse or children are in the examination room. It is perfectly proper for you to ask to be seen alone, without family in the room. It is also perfectly proper to voice your concerns and let the doctor know your symptoms, described in a way that is comfortable for you. The doctor can't help you if he doesn't know what is bothering you. Consultation with a urologist who specializes in male or female sexual dysfunction can be useful. If your sexual function has not been affected, there is no physical reason not to continue with a healthy sex life.

A Word about Exercise

Exercise will not cause further damage to nerves. In addition to providing electrical stimulation for the muscles to contract, nerve endings also release growth factors—chemicals that muscles need to stay healthy. Exercise will help keep your muscles as strong as they can be for as long as possible. Advice from a physical therapist is useful to make sure you are exercising properly.

A Word about Sleep

We all know that everything seems worse after a bad night's sleep. To get the best sleep you can, prepare for it. Take pain medication far enough in advance of bedtime to give it time to work. Avoid caffeine in the afternoon and evening. Limit alcohol consumption. Although a drink before bed can be relaxing and help you get to sleep, the effect of alcohol wears off after a few hours and can wake you up. Try not to nap during the day. Go to bed and wake up at the same time each day. Daily exercise, done early in the day, can lead to easier sleep at night. Exercise in the evening will be stimulating and may make it harder to fall asleep. Using local treatment, like a foot rub, a massaging foot bath, or a small amount of anesthetic ointment can also relieve pain long enough for you to fall asleep. My patients tell me they feel better in a cool room with light bedclothes.

Spend some time relaxing and clearing your mind before trying to fall asleep. A quiet room, calming music, and a good book can do wonders. And put the computer screens away! The bright light from the screen tells your brain that it is daytime, time to be awake. If you tend to awaken in the night with thoughts of all you have to do or worries about the day racing through your head, keep a pad of paper and a pen beside the bed to write down your thoughts so that you can stop thinking about them. A warm bath is a relaxing way to prepare for sleep. If your feet are cold, try heavy socks or socks that you heat in the microwave, being very careful not to make them too hot! Some people use ointments like Bengay to decrease foot pain before bed. These ointments can be irritating to sensitive skin and should not be used when there are breaks in the skin. A good night's sleep will help you better cope with the pain of neuropathy during the day.

I remember so clearly sitting in a doctor's office watching my husband fall asleep during a pinprick test. The doctor paused to look over at me, then said to my husband, "Do you feel anything?" My husband replied, "Tell me when you start." The diagnosis of neuropathy explained a lot: why my husband was too uncomfortable going out, why he would go to sleep to escape the burning cold feeling in his hands and feet, why I was always bandaging his second-degree burns from spilled coffee. Intimacy has a different meaning when one partner has injured nerves and the other is a caretaker. Neuropathy, with its overarching weakness and fatigue, has certainly changed our ways. It's about adapting—and adopting Plan B.

A book is a collaborative effort between those who inspire those who write, and those who edit, illustrate, and advise. I have been and continue to be inspired by my patients and their families who live with neuropathy. I am in awe of patients who have volunteered for clinical trials. I admire patients, families, health care providers, and others who educate and advocate through their research and through patient and family support groups.

Thank you to the following individuals and organizations for their inspiration, knowledge, and support in creating this book: my editor at Johns Hopkins University Press, Jacqueline Wehmueller, for guiding a first-timer through this process; Melanie Mallon, copyeditor, for making improvements to the text and preventing some embarrassment; Jane Whitney for her clear and accurate illustrations; Gene Taft, Kathy Alexander, Hilary Jacqmin, Juliana McCarthy, and the rest of the staff at Johns Hopkins University Press for editing, producing, and publicizing the book.

I thank Dr. Carlos Kase, chairman of neurology at Boston University School of Medicine, for his confidence, support, and guidance. I send great thanks to the Boston University Amyloidosis Treatment and Research Center, especially to Dr. John Berk, Dr. Martha Skinner, and the late Dr. David Seldin, for allowing me to care for patients with amyloid neuropathy for the past fifteen years.

It has been my privilege to work with the Amyloidosis Support Group. I send special appreciation to the group's founder and president, Muriel Finkel, for welcoming me into the fold. I thank the American Academy of Neurology and the American Association of Neuromuscular and Electrodiagnostic Medicine, who have been leaders in train-

...., advocates for the entire range of ... ...o provide patients and their families wit... ...d guidelines regarding the treatment of ne... ...part of a project spurred by advocacy training thro... ...cademy of Neurology.

...hank you to the many clinicians and researchers and th... ...ting organizations for research into the causes of and treat... ...t for neuropathy. In writing this book, I have relied on published ...ormation and guidelines from several organizations, including the ...merican Academy of Neurology, the American Association of Neuro- muscular and Electrodiagnostic Medicine, the American Diabetes As- sociation, and the Mayo Clinic.

A most special appreciation goes to my patients and their fami- lies at Boston University School of Medicine and at New York University School of Medicine, who were kind enough to share their experiences and thoughts, which are included in the book.

On a more personal note, I thank Dr. Marie Pasinski for showing me that this was something I could accomplish. You were my senior resident, and you lead me still. Love and gratitude go to my ultimate editors, my daughter, Hannah Jarmolowski; my husband, John Man- nion; and my mother, Myrtle Wiesman, for their patience, support, and multiple readings of the text. Finally, to my father, the late Myer Wies- man, for telling me I could do anything.

Glossary

acetylcholine A neurotransmitter that communicates between an axon and a muscle or sweat gland.

adrenaline A neurotransmitter released by autonomic nerves. Among other functions, it makes the heart beat faster. Another name for epinephrine.

adrenergic Referring to the system that uses adrenaline.

adrenomyeloneuropathy An inherited disorder that causes neuropathy and also affects the adrenal gland.

amyloidosis A general term referring to diseases that result from deposits of nonsoluble protein in tissues of the body. This is a cause of neuropathy.

aperture An opening that controls the amount of light that passes through a lens.

ataxia Inability to coordinate muscle movement. Also used to describe an uncoordinated gait.

atrophy Wasting and shrinkage. Used to describe the changes in muscle that occur with neuropathy.

autoimmune An immune system attack against the body itself.

autonomic Part of the nervous system that mediates automatic functions, such as heart rate, blood pressure, sweating, digestion, and sexual function.

autosomal Related to a chromosome other than a sex chromosome.

axial Relating to the trunk of the body.

axon The armlike extension produced by a neuron that reaches out to contact another neuron, muscle, or gland, or to bring sensory information back into the nervous system.

axonal Relating to an axon.

ayurvedic A form of alternative medicine that originated in India.

bariatric Related to the treatment of obesity, often used to refer to weight-loss surgery.

bilirubin A yellow-colored byproduct of hemoglobin breakdown that is found in bile and blood. High levels of bilirubin in the blood result in jaundice.

biopsy The removal of body tissue to examine for the purpose of diagnosis.

central nervous system The brain and spinal cord.

chelation The use of a chemical to bind with a metal in order to remove it from the body.

creatinine A byproduct of protein metabolism. Elevated blood levels are associated with kidney disease.

cryoglobulins Protein found in the blood that precipitates (separates from the blood) in cold temperature. May be related to infection with hepatitis C and may be a cause of neuropathy.

deciliter A tenth of a liter.

demyelinating Causing loss of the insulating fatty myelin coating around an axon.

dendrite Specialized endings of a neuron that bring information toward the neuron cell body.

diabetes mellitus An illness in which blood sugar is too high because of problems with the amount or function of insulin in the body.

dorsal Toward the back.

edema Swelling with fluid.

enteropathy Disease of the intestine.

enzyme A protein that facilitates normal chemical reactions in the body.

epinephrine A neurotransmitter; another name for adrenaline.

erythrocyte A red blood cell.

etiology The cause of a disease.

fasciculations Brief contractions of a small part of a muscle as a result of the random firing of a neuron or its axon. Occurs with damage to a neuron or axon.

ganglia A structure containing neurons.

gliadin One of many proteins that make up gluten.

gluten A protein found in wheat that has many subparts.

gray matter Part of the nervous system made up of neurons.

hemoglobin Oxygen-carrying protein found in red blood cells.

homeopathy A form of alternative medicine that treats disease by the administration of minute doses of a substance that would, in larger doses, produce symptoms of the disease.

homunculus A miniature person.

hypoglycemia Low blood sugar.

hypotension Low blood pressure.

hypothyroidism Low thyroid function resulting in a low level of thyroid hormone in the blood.

immunoglobulin A protein that is made by the immune system to fight off infection; also called an antibody.

inflammation A response to cell injury that involves white blood cells gathering around the damaged tissue as well as increased blood flow to the damaged area.

innervate To supply with nerves.

islet cell A specialized cell in the pancreas that produces insulin.

lacrimal Glands in the eyes that produce tears.

meninges The three membranes that surround the spinal cord and brain.

micron A unit of measure equal to one millionth of a meter.

myelin The fatty coating that surrounds and insulates axons.

neuron A cell that carries messages between the brain and other parts of the body. The basic unit of the nervous system.

neuropathy Generalized damage of nerves.

neurotransmitter A molecule that carries signals from one neuron to another neuron, muscle cell, or sweat gland.

norepinephrine A neurotransmitter.

oligodendrocyte Cell in the brain that makes the myelin surrounding axons in the central nervous system.

paraneoplastic Symptoms caused indirectly by the presence of cancer.

percutaneous Applied under the skin.

peripheral nervous system The part of the nervous system outside the brain and spinal cord. It consists of nerves, muscles, and sensory receptors.

radiculitis Inflammation of a nerve root.

radiculopathy Injury to a nerve as a result of it being damaged as it exits the spinal cord.

receptor A protein on the cell surface that has affinity for a specific molecule. When that molecule attaches to its receptor, it causes changes to take place in the cell.

Schwann cell Cell outside the brain and spinal cord that makes the myelin surrounding peripheral axons.

serotonin A neurotransmitter.

sorbitol A byproduct of glucose (sugar) metabolism.

sphincter muscle A ring-shaped muscle that closes down when it contracts.

stroke When a blood vessel in the brain is suddenly blocked, leading to loss of blood flow.

sudomotor Related to nerves that innervate sweat glands.

synapse The area at the end of an axon where a signal is transmitted from one neuron to another.

transcutaneous Applied to the surface of the skin.

uremia Accumulation in the blood of waste products that are usually excreted by the kidneys. A problem seen with kidney failure.

ventral Toward the front of the body.

vitamin Chemical consumed in the diet or made by the body that acts as a coenzyme, which enzymes require to carry out their chemical reactions in the body.

white matter Part of the central nervous system made up of axons.

References

p. 66, "The Diabetes Control and Complications Trial demonstrated": The Diabetes and Complications Trial Research Group. "The Effect of Intensive Diabetes Therapy on the Development and Progression of Neuropathy." *Annals of Internal Medicine* 122 (1995): 561–68.

p. 66, "In the study, this effect, to a lesser degree, continued": J. W. Albers et al. Diabetes Control and Complications Trial/Epidemiology of Diabetes Interventions and Complications Research Group. "Effect of Prior Intensive Insulin Treatment during the Diabetes Control and Complications Trial (DCCT) on Peripheral Neuropathy in Type 1 Diabetes during the Epidemiology of Diabetes Interventions and Complications (EDIC) Study." *Diabetes Care* 33 (2010): 1090–96.

p. 71, "Amitriptyline: a 10 to 25 mg tablet": Throughout the book I have relied on Medscape Reference (Reference.Medscape.com) for medication dosing recommendations.

p. 85, "Recent investigations in New York state": Anahad O'Connor. "New York Attorney General Targets Supplements at Major Retailers." Well blogs, *New York Times,* Feb. 3, 2015. http://well.blogs.nytimes.com/2015/02/03/new-york-attorney -general-targets-supplements-at-major-retailers

Resources

American Academy of Neurology
www.aan.com
Patient information regarding nervous system diseases

American Association of Neuromuscular and Electrodiagnostic Medicine
www.aanem.org
Patient information regarding neuropathy

American Diabetes Association
www.diabetes.org
Patient information regarding diabetes and neuropathy (available in English and Spanish)

Amyloidosis Support Groups
www.amyloidosissupport.org
Network of support groups around the United States for those with amyloidosis and their families

Charcot-Marie-Tooth Association
www.cmtausa.org
Information on inherited neuropathies

Family Caregiver Alliance
www.caregiver.org
Information, support, and advocacy for patient caregivers

Foundation for Peripheral Neuropathy
www.foundationforpn.org
Support and education for patients with neuropathy

GBS-CIPD Foundation International
www.gbs-cidp.org
Information on demyelinating neuropathies, such as Guillain-Barré syndrome (GBS) and chronic inflammatory demyelinating poly-neuropathy (CIDP)

Clinic

laxation techniques www.mayoclinic.org/healthy-lifestyle
/stress-management/basics/relaxation
-techniques/hlv-20049495

disease information www.mayoclinic.org/diseases-conditions
Patient-focused information in a variety of languages.

Muscular Dystrophy Association
www.mda.org
Information on inherited neuropathies

National Institute of Neurological Disorders and Stroke
www.ninds.nih.gov/
Coping with chronic pain (available in English and Spanish)

National Institutes of Health
health.nih.gov
General health information (available in English and Spanish)

National Library of Medicine's MedlinePlus
for consumer questions www.nlm.nih.gov/medlineplus
for medication information www.nlm.nih.gov/medlineplus/drug
information.html

National Center for Complementary and Integrative Health
www.nccih.nih.gov
*Educational resource for those interested in alternative medicine (available
in English and Spanish)*

PatientsLikeMe
www.patientslikeme.com
Networking for patients to connect with others who have the same illness

Index

acetaminophen, 73
acetylcholine, 69, 107
acid reflux, 81–82
action potentials, 2
acupuncture, 67
acute axonal neuropathy, 26, 32
acute inflammatory demyelinating
  polyneuropathy, 10
adrenaline, 8, 107, 108
adrenomyeloneuropathy, 26, 31, 107
AIDS. *See* human immunodeficiency
  virus (HIV) disease
alcohol use, 24, 35, 39, 96–97; acid reflux and, 82; blood pressure and, 77;
  limiting of, 64, 96, 100; opioid use
  and, 74; sleep and, 100; thiamine
  deficiency and, 29
α-blockers, 81
alpha-lipoic acid, 85
alprostadil penile injections, 83
alternative treatments, 84–85, 112
American Academy of Neurology, 46,
  69, 74, 111
American Association of
  Neuromuscular and
  Electrodiagnostic Medicine, 111
American Diabetes Association, 111
amitriptyline, 70–71
amyloid, 47
amyloidosis, 25, 26, 31, 52, 107
Amyloidosis Support Groups, 111
anatomy of nerves, 1–7

anesthesia dolorosa, 61
anesthetics, local, 68, 100; for bladder catheterization, 80; for lumbar
  puncture, 62; for nerve biopsy, 61;
  for nerve conduction studies/EMG,
  54–55; for skin biopsy, 60
anodyne light therapy, 84
antibiotics: for foot infections, 98, 99;
  neuropathy due to, 24, 34; for syphilis, 94
antibodies, 93, 109; in autoimmune diseases, 9, 10, 51; in cancer, 36, 47, 50; in
  celiac disease, 29; to hepatitis C, 32,
  50; to HIV, 49; in pernicious anemia,
  28; plasma exchange for removal of,
  11; postinfectious, 32
antidepressants: for bladder dysfunction, 81; for pain, 70–72
anti-inflammatory drugs, 73
antiseizure medications, 72
arm symptoms, 15, 18, 43; in metabolic
  diseases, 93; in multiple sclerosis, 93;
  occupational therapy for, 75, 97. *See
  also* hand/wrist symptoms
arsenic toxicity, 35, 67, 85
aspirin, 73
ataxia, 107; Friedreich's, 26, 31, 52
Ativan, 74
autoimmune disease, 9, 26, 30, 37, 51,
  92, 107
autoimmune neuropathy, 9–10, 26, 32,
  37, 51

autonomic functions, 2, 4, 14, 18; examination of, 44–45; testing of, 57–59
autonomic nerves, 2, 3–4, 5, 107
autonomic symptoms, 18–23, 40, 41; treatment of, 76–84
autosomal dominant inheritance, 11–12, 52
autosomal recessive inheritance, 12, 52
axonal length-dependent, dying-back neuropathy, 9, 10, 12–14; acute, 26, 32; treatment of, 13–14
axons, 1–2, 13, 107; autonomic, 5, 7; inherited disorders of, 11–12; motor, 3, 5, 7, 17; myelin coating of, 2, 3, 5, 7, 17, 109; neuropathy due to damage of, 24–25, 33; sensory, 3, 4, 5, 7; size and conduction speed of, 5, 7; small- and large-axon symptoms, 15–16, 43
Ayurvedic medicine, 85, 108

balance problems, 16, 40, 95; due to vitamin E deficiency, 29; examination of, 40, 43; physical therapy for, 75, 97
bariatric surgery, 28–29, 108
Bengay ointment, 100
benzocaine spray, 68
benzodiazepines, 74
bethanechol, 81
bilirubin, 93, 108
biopsy, 46, 60, 108; nerve, 55, 61; skin, 55, 60–61
bladder catheterization, 59, 79–81
bladder dysfunction, 18, 21–22, 40; testing for, 59; treatment of, 78–81
blood patch, 63
blood pressure, 4, 14, 18, 107; erectile dysfunction and, 83; exercise and, 75; lightheadedness and, 19, 76–77; low, 109; measurement of, 40, 44; medication-induced elevation of, 69, 71; during tilt table test, 57
blood pressure medications, 29, 30, 74
blood sugar (glucose): in diabetes mellitus, 25–27, 64–66, 93, 108; diet and,

81; exercise and, 75; fasting level, 25–26, 48; glucose intolerance and, 24; hemoglobin A1C and, 27, 49; high, 27, 49; low, 19, 23, 109; in prediabetes, 25–26; two-hour glucose tolerance test, 49
blood tests, 47–53, 73
blood thinners, 55
blood urea nitrogen, 48
blood vessels: alcohol effects on, 77; anodyne light therapy effects on, 84; arteries, 3, 18, 37; blood pressure, lightheadedness and, 19, 77; caffeine effects on, 63; in connective tissue diseases, 30; coronary, 23; in diabetes, 27; examination of, 40; inflammation of, 25, 37, 61; neuropathy due to damage of, 37; in penis, 22, 83; in rheumatologic diseases, 25; smoking effects on, 37, 97; stroke due to blockage of, 110
bone marrow cancer, 10, 31, 47, 50; neuropathy induced by medications for, 34
botulinum toxin injections: for pain, 68; for sweating, 78
bowel function, 4, 18, 19, 22
brain, 2–5; diseases of, 92
bugs-crawling-on-skin sensation, 8, 15
burning pain, 15, 40, 66, 69, 96, 101

caffeine: for post-lumbar puncture headache, 63; sleep and, 100
cancer, 10, 36–37, 47; neuropathy induced by medications for, 10–11, 14, 24–25, 33, 34, 84
cannabinoids, 67
carbamazepine, 72
caregiver support, 96, 111
carisoprodol (Soma), 72
carpal tunnel syndrome, 18, 91–92
causes of neuropathy, 24–37; amyloidosis, 31; blood vessel damage, 7; cancer, 36–37; celiac disease, 29; con-

nective tissue disease, 30; diabetes, 25–27; hypothyroidism, 31; in ICU, 30; illness, 24–25; infectious and postinfectious, 32; inherited metabolic illness, 31; kidney disease, 30–31; malnutrition, 28; medications, 33–35; toxins, 35–36; vitamin and mineral deficiency and toxicity, 28–29

celiac disease, 26, 29

central nervous system, 2, 108; diseases of, 92–93

cerebrospinal fluid, 62–63

Charcot-Marie-Tooth Association, 111

Charcot-Marie-Tooth disease, 11–12, 52

chelation therapy, 67, 108

chloroquine, 10

chromosomes, 11, 107

chronic inflammatory demyelinating polyneuropathy, 10, 26, 111

clinical trials, 86–89

coldness: of hands or feet, 15, 18, 19, 100, 101; sensation of, 4–5

complete blood count, 47

compression stockings, 77

computerized axial tomography (CT), 59–60

connective tissue diseases, 26, 30, 51

constipation, 22, 40, 82; medication-induced, 70, 71, 74

coordination problems, 16; ataxia, 107; due to vitamin E deficiency, 29; examination of, 40, 44; in tabes dorsalis, 94

copper excess, 29

cranial nerve examination, 41

creatinine, 48, 108

Credé maneuver, 79

cryoglobulins, 32, 50, 108

cyanocobalamin deficiency, 14, 26, 28–29, 47–48, 64

Data Safety and Review Board, 88

dehydration, 19, 74, 76, 77

demyelinating neuropathy, 9–11; autoimmune, 9–10; axonal, 10; vs. demyelinating central nervous system disease, 92–93; diagnosis of, 10; toxin-induced, 10; treatment of, 10–11

dendrites, 3, 108

desipramine, 70–71

Diabetes Control and Complications Trial, 66

diabetes mellitus, 23, 24, 25–27, 37, 108; blood sugar level/control in, 25–27, 64–66, 93, 108; carpal tunnel syndrome in, 91; erectile dysfunction in, 83; exercise in, 75; hemoglobin A1C in, 27, 49; mechanism of neuropathy in, 27; medications for neuropathy in, 69–70; skin biopsy in, 61; tests for, 47, 48–49, 53; treatment-related neuropathy in, 27; type 1 and type 2, 25; use of radiologic contrast agents in, 60

diagnosing neuropathy, 38–45; doctor-patient communication about, 45; medical history, 38–40; neurological examination, 40–45

diagnostic tests, 46–63; autonomic function tests, 57–59; blood tests, 47–53; CT and MRI, 59–60; doctor-patient communication about, 63; ECG, 53; lumbar puncture, 62–63; nerve biopsy, 61; nerve conduction studies and EMG, 53–55; quantitative sensory testing, 55–56; skin biopsy, 60–61; ultrasound, 57; urine tests, 53

dialysis, 30–31

diarrhea, 22, 32, 40; treatment of, 82

diet/nutrition, 97; alcohol in, 35, 64; for diabetes, 23, 66; dietary supplements, 85; for gastrointestinal symptoms, 81–82; high-fiber, 82; lightheadedness and, 77; malnutrition, 14, 22, 26, 28, 30; sensitivity to gluten in, 29; vitamins and minerals in, 28–29, 110

diphenoxylate/atropine, 82
diphtheria, 10, 32
double-blind, randomized placebo-
  controlled trials, 87
driving, 91, 97
droxidopa, 77
dry eyes, 18, 20, 40, 70
dry mouth, 14, 18, 20, 40; medication-
  induced, 70, 71, 72, 82
dry skin, 18, 20, 98
duloxetine, 70, 71

edema, 17, 108
electrical sensations, 8, 15, 16
electrocardiogram (ECG), 53, 73
electromyography (EMG), 53–55
EMLA cream, 68
enteropathy, 108; gluten-sensitive, 29
enzymes, 28, 108; digestive, 20; liver, 50;
  in porphyria, 52; vitamins as coenzymes, 28, 110
erectile dysfunction, 14, 22, 40, 70;
  treatment of, 82–83
erythrocytes, 51, 108
erythrocyte sedimentation rate, 51
esomeprazole (Nexium), 75
etiologic treatment, 64–65
etiology, 108; of neuropathy, 24–37.
  See also causes of neuropathy
exercise, 15, 19, 75–76, 97, 99; in diabetes, 75; sleep and, 100
eyes, 18, 21; adjustment to light, 78; in
  diabetes, 66; dry, 18, 20, 40, 70; examination of, 41, 44; lacrimal glands
  in, 18, 20, 109

Fabry disease, 26, 31
fainting, 19, 53, 58, 76. See also lightheadedness
falls, 19, 70, 76, 97
Family Caregiver Alliance, 111
fasciculations (twitching), 15, 17, 42,
  72, 108

fatigue, 8, 15, 101
fludrocortisone, 77
Foley catheter, 80
foot/ankle symptoms, 8, 16, 18; alternative treatments for, 84; coldness, 19,
  100, 101; deformities, 17, 45, 98; driving and, 97; due to radiculopathy,
  90; due to vitamin deficiencies, 28,
  29; falls due to, 97; massage for, 66,
  100; in multiple sclerosis, 93; muscle
  weakness, 17–18, 45, 69, 97, 98; after
  nerve biopsy, 61; physical therapy
  for, 75; sensory, 42, 43, 45, 56, 97; topical lidocaine for, 68; ulcers, 98
foot care, 98–99
foot examination/inspection, 40, 45,
  95, 98
Foundation for Peripheral Neuropathy,
  111
Friedreich's ataxia, 26, 31, 52

gabapentin, 72
gait training, 75, 97
gallbladder disease, 93
ganglia, 3, 109; dorsal root, 30
gastrointestinal symptoms, 18, 22;
  treatment of, 81–82
GBS-CIPD Foundation International, 111
Genetic Information Nondiscrimination
  Act, 53
genetic mutations, 11–12; testing for,
  11, 52–53
gliadin, 29, 109
glossary, 107–10
gluten, 29, 108
Guillain-Barré syndrome, 10, 26, 32, 111

hair loss, 18, 20; thallium-induced,
  35, 36
hair toxin screening, 51
hand/wrist symptoms, 8, 15, 18; assistive devices for, 97–98; in carpal tunnel syndrome, 18, 91–92; coldness,

15, 18, 19, 101; driving and, 97; due to
vitamin deficiencies, 28, 29; motor,
17; muscle weakness, 15, 17–18, 97;
occupational therapy for, 75, 76, 97;
sensory, 16, 43
headache: in hypoglycemia, 23; after
lumbar puncture, 62–63; medication-induced, 72, 81
heart attack, 19, 66; silent, 23
heart rate, 2, 4, 18, 45, 107; ECG and,
53; lightheadedness and, 19; low
blood sugar and, 23; during tilt table
test, 57
heart rate deep breathing, 58–59
heavy metal toxicity, 35; chelation therapy for, 67, 108; screening for, 51
hemoglobin, 49, 109; A1C, 27, 49; in
porphyria, 51
hepatitis C, 26, 32, 50, 108
hereditary sensory-motor neuropathy
type I, 11–12
herpes zoster, 90–91
home modifications, 76
homeopathy, 85, 109
homunculus, 2, 3, 4, 109
human immunodeficiency virus (HIV)
disease, 26, 32; cannabinoids in, 67;
neuropathy induced by medications
for, 33, 34; test for, 49
Human Subjects Institutional Review
Board, 88
hypoglycemia, 23, 109
hypotension, 109; orthostatic (see lightheadedness)
hypothyroidism, 26, 31, 109

illness-associated neuropathy, 24–26.
See also specific diseases
imaging studies: CT and MRI, 59–60;
ultrasound, 57
immunoglobulin, 109. See also antibodies
infectious causes, 9, 10, 26, 32

inflammation, 51, 109; of blood vessels, 25, 37, 61; in celiac disease, 29;
of nerve roots, 90, 110; of sensory
nerves in herpes zoster, 91; of stomach, 28
informed consent for clinical trial par-
ticipation, 87–88, 89
inherited neuropathy, 9, 11–12, 26, 31;
testing for, 52–53
innervation, 109; by autonomic nerves,
4, 19–21, 61, 77; of muscles, 3, 17, 21,
42, 77; of sweat glands, 20, 61, 78, 110;
of vagina, 83
insulin, 25, 108, 109
intensive care unit (ICU), 30
intravenous immunoglobulin, 10
Islet cells of pancreas, 25, 109
itching, 15, 93

joint position sense, 7, 14, 94; testing
of, 43, 44

kidney disease, 78, 93, 108, 110; chelation therapy and, 67; medication
dosage and, 72; neuropathy due to,
26, 30–31; tests for, 47, 48, 53; use of
radiologic contrast agents in, 60

laboratory tests. See diagnostic tests
lansoprazole (Prevacid), 75
lead toxicity, 35, 67, 85
leg braces, 75
leg symptoms, 15, 18; due to radiculopathy, 90; falls due to, 97; after lumbar
puncture, 62; in metabolic diseases,
93; in multiple sclerosis, 93; muscle
weakness, 17–18, 42, 92, 93, 97; sensory, 16, 43; sweating, 20; swelling,
17, 72; in syphilis, 94. See also foot/
ankle symptoms
leprosy, 25, 26, 32
lidocaine, topical, 68
lifestyle changes, 63, 76, 82, 96–97

lightheadedness, 14, 18, 19, 40; antidepressant-induced, 70; driving and, 97; ECG for, 53; during heart rate deep breathing, 58; during tilt table test, 57–58; treatment of, 76–77
linolenic acid, 85
liver function tests, 50
living with neuropathy, 95–101; driving, 97; exercise, 99; falls, 19, 70, 76, 97; foot care, 98–99; lifestyle changes, 63, 76, 82, 96–97; sexuality, 99; sleep, 100–101; support groups, 96, 111–12; use of hands, 97–98
loperamide, 82
lumbar puncture, 62–63
Lyme disease, 50, 90

magnesium supplements, 75–76
magnetic resonance imaging (MRI), 59–60
malnutrition, 14, 22, 26, 28, 30
marijuana smoking, 67
massage, foot, 66, 100
Mayo Clinic, 112
medical history, 38–40
medication-induced neuropathy, 10, 16, 24, 26, 33–35
meninges, 6, 109
mental status examination, 41
mercury toxicity, 35, 51, 67, 85
metabolic diseases, 26, 31; inherited, 26, 31; vs. peripheral neuropathy, 93. *See also* diabetes mellitus
metoclopramide, 81
midodrine, 77
mononeuropathy, 8
motor nerves, 2–3, 5, 6, 17
motor symptoms, 16–18; examination of, 42; treatment of, 74–76
multiple sclerosis, 67, 92–93
muscle(s): atrophy of, 17, 42, 98, 107; diseases of, 92; fasciculations of, 15, 17, 42, 72, 108; innervation of, 3, 17, 21, 42, 77

muscle cramps, 8, 15, 17; treatment of, 74–75
muscle relaxers, 72
muscle weakness, 11, 14, 15, 16–18, 40, 65, 74, 95, 101; botulinum toxin–induced, 69; in carpal tunnel syndrome, 91; driving and, 97; due to lead exposure, 25; due to radiculopathy, 90; due to vitamin deficiencies, 29; in feet, 17–18, 45, 69, 97, 98; in hands, 15, 17–18, 97; in multiple sclerosis, 93; in muscle diseases, 92; pattern of, 42; radiation-induced, 36; vs. sensory loss, 18; testing for, 42
Muscular Dystrophy Association, 112
myelin coating of axons, 2, 3, 5, 7, 17, 109; inherited disorders of, 11–12; medication-induced damage of, 24, 33; in multiple sclerosis, 92; neuropathy due to damage of, 9–11

nabiximols, 67
nails, 18, 20, 95; filing/trimming of, 95, 98
naproxen, 73
narcotics for pain, 73–74, 96
National Center for Complementary and Integrative Health, 112
National Institutes of Health, 112
National Institutes of Neurological Disorders and Stroke, 112
National Library of Medicine's MedlinePlus, 112
nerve(s): autonomic, 2, 3–4, 5; blood supply to, 37; definition of, 1; emergence from spinal cord, 5; motor, 2–3, 5, 17; percutaneous stimulation of, 66–67; regeneration of, 13–14, 16, 64; sensory, 2, 3, 4–5
nerve biopsy, 55, 61
nerve conduction studies (NCS), 53–55
nerve roots, 2, 5, 6
Neuracel, 85
neurological examination, 40–45

neuron(s), 1–2, 109; axons supported by, 13; cell body of, 1, 2, 13
neuropathy, 8, 109; autoimmune, 9–10, 26, 32, 37, 51; axonal, 9, 10, 12–14; causes of, 24–37; conditions that feel like, 90–94; demyelinating, 9–11; diagnosis of, 38–45; inherited, 9, 11–12, 26, 31; living with, 95–101; support groups for, 96, 111–12; symptoms of, 8, 15–23; treatment of, 64–85; types of, 9–14
neurotransmitters, 1–2, 3, 70, 83, 109
Nexium (esomeprazole), 75
nicotine, 37, 96–97
nitrous oxide, 83
norepinephrine, 70, 109
nortriptyline, 70–71
numbness, 8, 15, 16, 35, 40, 66, 92, 95, 96; in carpal tunnel syndrome, 91; due to radiculopathy, 90; in hands, 97; in multiple sclerosis, 93; after nerve biopsy, 61; radiation-induced, 36

occupational therapy, 75–76, 95–96, 97
oligodendrocytes, 92, 109
omeprazole (Prilosec), 75
opioids for pain, 73–74, 96
organophosphate insecticide exposure, 36

pain, 8, 14, 15–16, 39, 43, 95; abdominal, 22, 51; in amyloidosis, 31; in carpal tunnel syndrome, 91; in connective tissue diseases, 30; due to thallium exposure, 35; due to vitamin deficiencies, 28, 29; falls due to, 97; in hands, 97; of heart attack, 23; heat that feels like, 56; after initiation of diabetes treatment, 27; lightning, in syphilis, 94; loss of ability to feel, 98; of lumbar puncture, 62; of muscle cramps, 17; in muscle diseases, 92; after nerve biopsy, 61; of nerve

conduction studies/EMG, 54–55; in paraneoplastic neuropathy, 36; in porphyria, 51; of radiculopathy, 90; sensation of, 4, 7; sexual effects of, 82, 83; sleep and, 97, 100. See also specific types of pain
pain medications, 68–74, 96; antidepressants, 70–72; anti-inflammatory drugs, 73; antiseizure drugs, 72; before bedtime, 100; opioid, 73–74, 96; topical, 67–68
pain treatment, 65–66; alternative treatments, 84–85; botulinum toxin injections, 68; clinical trials, 86; marijuana, 67; without medication, 66–67; medications, 68–74, 96; topical anesthetics, 67–68
papaverine with alprostadil penile injections, 83
paraneoplastic neuropathy, 26, 36–37, 110
PatientsLikeMe, 112
percutaneous nerve stimulation, 66–67
perhexiline, 10
peripheral nervous system, 2, 92, 110
pernicious anemia, 28
phentolamine with alprostadil penile injections, 83
phenytoin, 72
physical examination, 40
physical therapy, 75–76, 96, 97, 99
polyneuropathy, 8; acute inflammatory demyelinating, 10; chronic inflammatory demyelinating, 10, 26, 111
Pompe disease, 26, 31, 52
porphyria, 26, 31; tests for, 51–52
postinfectious neuropathy, 26, 32
prediabetes, 24, 25, 27. See also diabetes mellitus
pregabalin, 70, 72
pressure sensation, 4, 7
Prevacid (lansoprazole), 75
Prilosec (omeprazole), 75
procainamide, 10

proton-pump inhibitors, 74–75
pyridoxine excess or deficiency, 14, 26,
    28, 29, 34, 47–48, 64–65, 85

quantitative sensory testing (QST),
    55–56
quantitative sudomotor axon reflex
    test (QSART), 58
quinine, 75

radiculitis, 90–91, 110
radiculopathy, 90–91, 110
rapid plasma reagin (RPR) test, 49
receptors, 1–4, 110
regeneration of nerves, 13–14, 16, 64
relaxation techniques, 100, 112
resources, 111–12
rheumatoid arthritis, 25, 26, 30, 34
Romberg maneuver, 43

Schwann cells, 2, 5, 92, 110
sedatives, 72
selective serotonin and norepineph-
    rine reuptake inhibitors (SSNRIs):
    for bladder dysfunction, 81; for pain,
    70, 71
sensation testing, 56
sensory examination, 42–43; QST, 55–56
sensory neurons, 2, 3, 4–5, 6
sensory symptoms, 15–16; negative
    and positive, 15, 66; small- and large-
    axon, 15–16, 43; treatment of, 65–74;
    vs. weakness, 18
serotonin, 70, 110
serum protein electrophoresis and im-
    munofixation, 49
sexual dysfunction, 14, 18–19, 22, 40,
    82, 99; antidepressant-induced, 70;
    treatment in men, 82–83; treatment
    in women, 83–84
shingles, 91
shooting pain, 15, 94
sildenafil, 83

Sjögren's disease, 26, 30, 51
skin: dry, 18, 20, 98; sensitivity of, 2, 3,
    4, 7, 15–16
skin biopsy, 55, 60–61
sleep problems, 8, 40, 91, 97, 100–101;
    elevating head of bed for, 76, 82;
    pain medications and, 66, 70, 73, 74
smell sense, 5, 20, 41
smoking: marijuana, 67; tobacco, 27, 37,
    39, 96–97
Soma (carisoprodol), 72
sorbitol, 27, 110
spinal cord, 2–6; diseases of, 92
spinal nerves, 6
spinal tap, 62–63
squeezing sensation, 15, 40
stiffness, 15, 16
strength testing, 42
stroke, 25, 66, 110
sudomotor nerves, 58, 110
support groups, 96, 111–12
sweating, 18, 20, 107; antidepressant-
    induced, 70, 71; of feet, 98; low blood
    sugar and, 23; management of, 78;
    on QSART, 58
symptoms, 8, 15–23; autonomic, 18–23;
    history of, 40; limitations due to,
    15; motor, 16–18, 42; sensory, 15–16,
    42–43; small- and large-axon, 15–16,
    43; treatment of, 64–85
synapse, 1, 3, 110
syphilis, 49, 93–94
systemic lupus erythematosus, 25, 26,
    30, 51

tabes dorsalis, 94
tacrolimus, 10
tadalafil, 83
tai chi, 75
tamsulosin hydrochloride, 81
taste sense, 16, 41
temperature sensation, 4–5, 7; testing
    of, 56

tendon reflex testing, 43–44
terazosin, 81
thallium exposure, 35
thiamine deficiency, 26, 28, 29, 47
thyroid disease, 65, 91; hypothyroidism, 26, 31, 109; tests for, 47, 48
thyroid hormone, 31, 48, 109
tilt table test, 57–58
tincture of opium, 82
tingling, 15, 16, 36, 40, 90, 92, 96; in carpal tunnel syndrome, 91; in metabolic diseases, 93; treatment of, 65, 66, 68, 69
tocopherol deficiency, 29
touch sensation, 4, 7, 15–16; testing of, 56
toxic neuropathy, 10, 24, 26, 35–36
toxoid injections, 10
transcutaneous electric nerve stimulation (TENS), 67
transthyretin, 31
treatment, 64–85; alternative, 84–85, 112; of autonomic symptoms, 76–84; of axonal neuropathy, 13–14; clinical trials, 86–89; of demyelinating neuropathy, 10–11; etiologic vs. symptomatic, 64–65; future, 84; of motor symptoms, 74–76; of sensory symptoms, 65–74
tricyclic antidepressants, 70–71
triglycerides, 27
tuning fork test, 43, 56

ultrasound, 57
urea, 48, 93

uremia/uremic neuropathy, 26, 31, 110
urine tests, 53, 73
U.S. Food and Drug Administration (FDA), 67, 69, 71, 72, 75, 85, 87, 88

vaccinations, 10
vaginal dryness, 83
Valium, 74
Valsalva maneuver, 79, 110
vardenafil, 83
venlafaxine, 71
vertebral column, 3, 6
vibration sense, 4, 7, 8; testing of, 43, 56
vision symptoms, 18, 21, 40, 78
vitamin/mineral deficiencies or toxicity, 26, 28–29; copper, 29; testing for, 47–48; vitamin B1, 26, 28, 29, 47; vitamin B6, 14, 26, 28, 29, 34, 47–48, 64–65, 85; vitamin B12, 14, 26, 28–29, 47–48, 64; vitamin E, 29
vitamins, 28, 110

walking aids, 97
walking problems, 11, 15, 17; examination of, 40, 44; falls due to, 97; gait training for, 75, 97; physical therapy for, 75; in untreated syphilis, 94
weight-loss surgery, 28–29, 108

Xanax, 74
X-linked inheritance, 12, 52

yoga, 75

zimelidine, 10